COMPLETE VORTEX CONTROL SELF-DEFENSE

HAND TO HAND COMBAT, KNIFE DEFENSE, AND STICK FIGHTING

SAM FURY

Illustrated by
NEIL GERMIO, GIACOMO PILATO, AND ELIANA BASTIDA

Copyright SF Nonfiction Books © 2017

www.SFNonfictionBooks.com

All Rights Reserved
No part of this document may be reproduced without written consent from the author.

This publication has the approval of Peter Sunbye, creator of Vortex Control Self-Defense.

WARNINGS AND DISCLAIMERS

The information in this publication is made public for reference only.

Neither the author, publisher, nor anyone else involved in the production of this publication is responsible for how the reader uses the information or the result of his/her actions.

CONTENTS

Introduction	ix
Explanation of Terms	1
Principles of Self-Defense	3

PART I
HAND TO HAND COMBAT

Stepping	17
Weight Distribution Drill	19
Bombs	21
Bouncing Kicks	25

ENTRIES

Slap Entries	29
Thrust Entries	36
Curve Entries	39
Contact Entries	42
Rib Entries	44
Hand Formula	46
Lock Flow Drill	51

PART II
KNIFE DEFENSE

Attack	71
Defense	73
Knife Stepping Drills	78
Group A	83
Group B	87
Group C	92
Group D	96
Breaks	100
Universals	108

Self-Kills	115
Knife Flow Drill	119

BONUS CHAPTERS

Improvised Weapons	127
Weapon Vs Weapon	133

PART III
STICK FIGHTING

Explanation of Terms	137
Basic Stance	139
Stepping	140
The King of Strikes	141
Queen Strike	145
Strike Drills	148
Abanico Defense	155
Stick Parries	156
Defense Drill	159
Snatches	160
Grab and Strike Drills	177
Grab and Strike Defense Drills	193
Break-Outs	204
Double-Grab Scenarios	207
References	215
Author Recommendations	217
About Sam Fury	219

THANKS FOR YOUR PURCHASE

Did you know you can get FREE chapters of any SF Nonfiction Book you want?

https://offers.SFNonfictionBooks.com/Free-Chapters

You will also be among the first to know of FREE review copies, discount offers, bonus content, and more.

Go to:

https://offers.SFNonfictionBooks.com/Free-Chapters

Thanks again for your support.

INTRODUCTION

In this self-defense training manual, Sam Fury puts Vortex Control Self-Defense lessons learned in the Philippines onto paper.

Vortex Control Self-Defense is a unique fighting system created by Peter Sunbye. To create this system of self-defense, Peter traveled for 20+ years, searching for "lost" self-defense techniques.

He combined a number of martial arts, including GM Lawrence Lee's Tong Kune Do kung fu, Wing Chun, Balintawak Arnis Escrima, and Panatukan to create a highly effective and relatively easy to learn self-defense system. Once the basics are learned, Vortex Control Self-Defense can be applied effectively by almost anyone, regardless of their dexterity, strength, or fitness level.

This volume combines the three Vortex Control Self-Defense training manuals into one. It is presented in three parts.

Hand-to-Hand Combat

Covers everything to do with Vortex Control Self-Defense hand-to-hand combat.

Practical Escrima Knife Defense

Knife defense is the ability to defend yourself against an attacker who has a knife, though the techniques used can be applied to many other weapon attacks.

Knife fighting is extremely dangerous. In real life, it must be avoided at all costs. Never expect to go into a knife fight and come out unharmed. Even if you "win," you'll probably get cut, or worse. Be sure to use a training knife when practicing the techniques described here.

Practical Arnis Stick-Fighting

Kali Arnis is a Filipino martial art based on stick-fighting. This book combines methods learnt from a variety of Kali Arnis grandmasters and focuses on highly practical stick-fighting techniques and training drills.

This publication has been written under the approval of Peter Sunbye.

EXPLANATION OF TERMS

A few terms are used throughout this book to help describe the flow of movement.

Lead/Rear Side

Your lead side is whichever side of your body is forward-most and your rear side is whichever side of your body is rear-most. For example, if you're in a right-foot-forward stance, then your right side is your lead side, and your left side is your rear side.

Inside/Outside of Your Opponent's Guard

When your opponent's guard is up, you can place your arm either inside or outside of it.

Being inside your opponent's guard means that your limb is in between his limbs, closer to his center. Your arm is sandwiched by his.

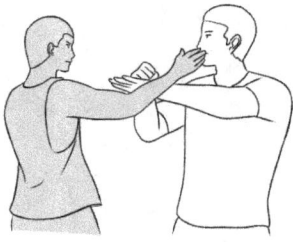

Being outside your opponent's guard means your opponent's limbs are both to either the left or right of your limb.

The pictures demonstrate being inside/outside of your opponent's guard with your arms, but it also applies to your legs. That is, you need to step to the outside of your opponent's guard in order to get behind him.

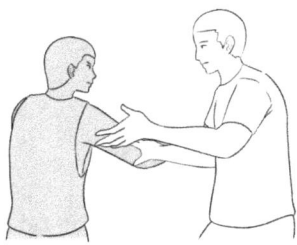

Just as you can be inside or outside your opponent's guard, he can be inside/outside yours.

Guarding Your Opponent's Limb

The expression "to guard your opponent's limb" means to put your limb close or on his limb so that you can't be struck by it. It is a pre-emptive defensive maneuver that may also be referred to as "covering your opponent's limb."

Throughout this book, the word "limb" is replaced as appropriate. For example, in the previous picture the man is using his right hand to guard/cover the woman's right elbow.

PRINCIPLES OF SELF-DEFENSE

The following principles are the core of Vortex Control Self-Defense. Although explained in reference to hand-to-hand combat, they are also applicable to weaponry.

Without these principles, the rest of this book is just a bunch of techniques that you can mimic. With them, the techniques in this book become a collection of examples of how the principles can be applied. You can then replicate techniques and/or create customized to ones.

The Vortex Control Self-Defense principles are all of equal importance, and are presented here in alphabetical order.

Constant Barrage

In Vortex Control Self-Defense there, you are constantly slapping, twisting, pulling, and pushing your opponent. This serves at least one (and usually several, if not all) of the following purposes:

- It confuses and disorients your opponent.
- It often lets you move your opponent one way while striking from the opposite direction. This increases the force of your strike.
- The movements in themselves bring a certain degree of discomfort and pain.
- It lets you place your opponent in the ideal position for your next move.

This also makes use of Newton's first law of motion, which states that:

> "An object at rest stays at rest, and an object in motion stays in motion with the same speed and in the same direction unless acted upon by an unbalanced force."

In reference to your movement, this means that it's better for you to keep moving once you're in motion. This is because it takes more energy to stop and restart than it does to continue an existing motion. In addition, the continued motion will be faster and therefore more powerful than if you were to start from inertia.

Counters

In martial arts, a counter is an attack made in response to your opponent's attack. It is about being proactive.

There is always a counter to your opponent's move, and there is a counter to your counter, and a counter to that counter. It can go on forever. The victor will be whoever has the foresight and/or intuition to out-counter their opponent.

Close combat is a game of chess. Fast chess. Instinctive chess.

Note: The closer you get to your opponent, the fewer opportunities there are for counters. You can use this to your advantage by first closing distance while gaining an advantageous position, and then finishing the fight before your opponent recovers.

Grounding

Grounding yourself means being in solid contact with the ground.

When you're grounded, you have more stability, and can therefore generate more powerful attacks. Power in strikes comes up from the ground. This is a well-known concept in the world of martial arts.

A simple exercise you can do to get the feeling of grounding is to pretend that you're drilling your body into the ground.

Grounding in this way is also well demonstrated in the weight distribution drill.

The act of grounding can also be used to increase damage by letting gravity do the work. This is well demonstrated in angulated stepping and the bomb-kick.

To get the feeling of using grounding in this manner, lift both your legs off the ground without jumping. Just let gravity do its thing.

Fulcrums

Body mechanics, paired with physics, play a big part in the efficiency of Vortex Control Self-Defense. By using parts of your body as fulcrums, you can gain more leverage, apply locks, break limbs, etc.

One-Handed Fighting

Both arms are used in the demonstrations in this book, but the unarmed portion of Vortex Control Self-Defense is developed so that most of the techniques can be done one-handed. This becomes extremely useful in real-life scenarios, such as when you are holding something you can't drop, like a baby, or when your arm gets injured. Once you have a good grasp of the techniques, you should train to do them with one hand. Just don't use your rear hand.

Power Angles

This is another principle based on physics and body mechanics.

There are certain angles that create the strongest frames. Your limbs should never be below 120° or above 160°.

120° is best for defense. Any smaller of an angle, and your arm will easily collapse when it's pushed towards you.

160° is best for attack. Any larger of an angle, and your arm can be easily pushed to the side. Holding it at an angle greater than 160° will also make it more susceptible to being captured—by being placed in a lock, for example.

As a rule, keep your limb at 120°. When you strike, extend it to 160° and then let your body push through. This combines power angles with grounding. Add in spring-loading and aim for the spine and you have the ideal the Vortex Control Self-Defense strike.

Spine Center

The Spine Center principle is based on the centerline theory, which is common in many martial arts, including Wing Chun. To explain the concept, here is an excerpt from the book *Basic Wing Chun Training* by Sam Fury:

www.SFNonfictionBooks.com/Basic-Wing-Chun-Training

Your centerline is an imaginary line drawn vertically down the center of your body. All the vital organs are located near the center of the body. Keep it away from your opponent by angling it away from him/her.

Controlling the position of your centerline in relation to your opponent's is done with footwork. Understanding the centerline will allow you to instinctively know where your opponent is.

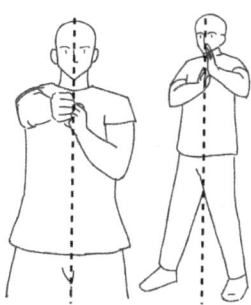

Your central line (different from your centerline) is drawn from your angled center to your opponent.

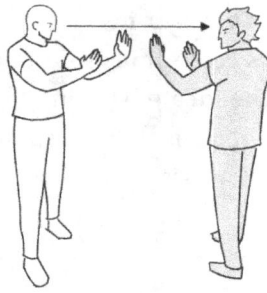

Offensively, you generate the most power when punching out from your center, since you can incorporate your whole body and hips.

When you're attacking in a straight line, your centerline should face away from your opponent, while your central line faces his/her center.

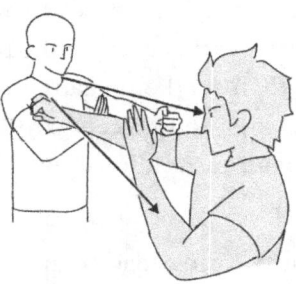

With hook punches and other circular attacks, the center- and central lines merge.

There are three main guidelines for the centerline.

- The one who controls the centerline will control the fight.
- Protect and maintain your own centerline while you control and exploit your opponent's.
- Control the centerline by occupying it.

In Vortex Control Self-Defense, instead of putting your offensive focus on your opponent's centerline as described above, focus on his spine. Doing so makes the idea of striking through your target more intuitive. An added advantage is that his spine can be affected by the many jerks, twists, etc. that are commonly used in Vortex Control Self-Defense.

Spring-Loading

Yet another principle based on the combination of body mechanics and physics is spring-loading.

The basic premise is that your muscles can be pushed in like a spring. These springs are then released in strikes, increasing speed and therefore power.

Speed in strikes is not just about how fast you reach the target. You must also be quick to recover. Recovery is the process of reloading the spring, which you can then send out again. In your arm, your triceps are the spring forward and your biceps are the spring back. Alternating spring-loading your arms allows you to make multiple strikes in very quick succession.

You can and should also spring-load your legs. The groin kick is a clear demonstration of this, but the motion should be present in all your movements.

It's important to remain relaxed. The spring is loaded and released, but never tensed so much that it slows you down.

Taking Space

Always crowd your opponent. Get in his space and claim it. Constantly push him back, and don't let up. This will unbalance him both mentally and physically.

Following the Thank You Principle

Take whatever your opponent gives you and use it to your advantage. If he applies pressure in a particular direction, flow with it. Redirect it if needed, but don't directly oppose it.

Those that want to become really good at this are encouraged to practice Chi Sao. Although live instruction is always preferred, the book *How to do Chi Sao* by Sam Fury is highly recommended.

www.SFNonfictionBooks.com/Chi-Sao

Another use of the thank you principle is to always take something back. For example, when retracting your limb from a strike, grab your opponent's arm or nose-ring.

Vibrating

In Vortex Control Self-Defense, the principle of vibrating is used to enhance the effectiveness of movement. It can be applied in many situations, such as when you're increasing the force in locks, making repetitive strikes, escaping holds, etc.

The following examples offer safe demonstrations of the effectiveness of vibrating:

The first example is a shirt-grab escape. Say an attacker grabs you by the shirt-front. Reach over his arms and grab his right wrist. At the same time, use your left hand to grab the same arm.

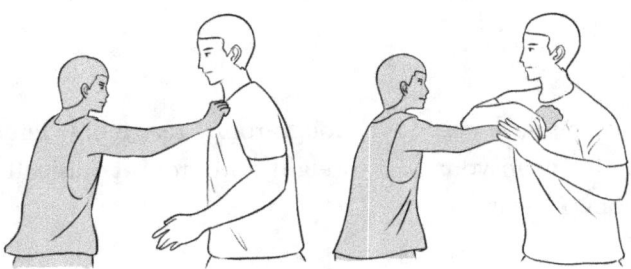

To release your opponent's grip, twist your body to your right using a waterfall motion.

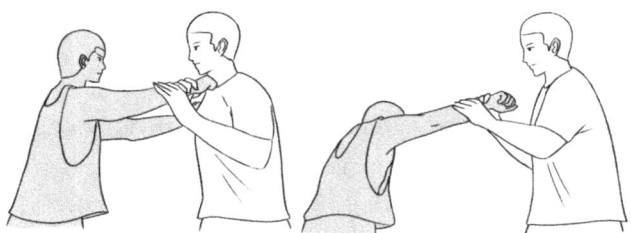

This move itself is a common and effective self-defense technique, but when your attacker is much stronger than you, it may not work. Increase its effectiveness by vibrating.

As you twist your body, make small, fast, jerking movements. Concentrate these movements into your twisting motion, especially where your opponent is gripping you.

The next example is a rear bear hug escape. Say an attacker puts you in a rear bear hug with your arms pinned. A common way to get out of this is with rear elbows, but if your opponent's grip is too tight, you won't have the room to do this. Vibrate your body to create space.

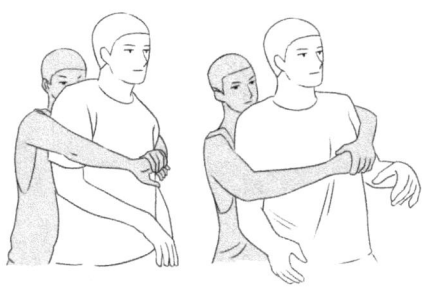

As soon as you have even just enough room, rear elbow left and then right. Finally, drop your body weight and ground yourself to break your opponent's grip.

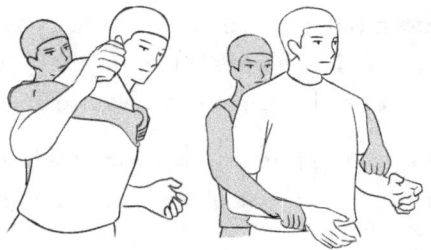

Vortex

By using the motion of a vortex (like water going down a sinkhole) you can easily break through your opponent's defense. For example, if your opponent is pushing your hand in a certain direction, you can use a vortex motion to move under and around it. This is actually the basis of the curve entry.

Another way to use the vortex is if your opponent grabs your arm. A fast vortex motion will most likely free you from his grip while you counter-strike in the same motion. In most cases, you'll want to vortex towards your opponent's spine.

Warfare Strategy

The strategy for attack in Vortex Control Self-Defense mimics that of warfare.

Intelligence. First, you must gather intelligence so you can make the right decision regarding your enemy. In warfare, this is done through methods such as espionage. In self-defense, it's better understood as "sizing up" your opponent.

Within a few seconds of studying your enemy, you can determine any weaknesses he has (such as obvious injuries), sense his fear (or lack thereof), assess his ability (speed, strength, skill), etc. You can also assess your surroundings and identify possible escape routes, available weapons, etc.

Bombs. After your initial assessment, assuming you feel that fighting is necessary, attack with bombs. The military uses planes and mortars. In Vortex Control Self-Defense, we use bomb-kicks.

Infantry. Finally, once the bombs have done their job, the infantry is sent in. This translates to the use of entry techniques and the fighting formula.

Waterfall

The analogy of water going over the edge of a waterfall is often used to explain how to perform certain movements used in the techniques. The free-fall of water is also akin to grounding. Combing the three actions of waterfall, grounding, and vortex is extremely powerful.

Weaponizing

The principle of weaponizing means to make as many of your movements as much like attacks as possible, even if they are primarily defensive or neutral. Here are some examples:

- Instead of just placing your foot down after a kick, stomp your opponent's knee or foot.
- When defending against an incoming strike, don't just block it. Instead, block it in a way that hurts your opponent as well. Punch his arm (a stop-hit), for example.
- Your intention may be to apply a lock, but you can make various strikes in the process.
- After hitting your opponent, hit him again while retracting your limb.

Yin and Yang

The well-known Chinese Taoism concept of yin and yang is also applied in Vortex Control Self-Defense, where yin is "soft" and yang is "hard."

Soft does not equal weak, and it is the combination of soft and hard, fast and slow, light and heavy (grounded), etc. that will make your techniques work together.

Here are some examples to demonstrate the use of yin and yang in the context of Vortex Control Self-Defense. These are just a few examples of a concept that applies to everything in the universe.

- Tai Chi is very yin (slow and soft) in practice, and to the layman it may seem useless for combat, but if you speed the movements up to become yang (hard and fast), they can be devastating.
- In training, it's useful to use more yin and less yang. Doing things slowly (yin) first allows your mind and body to "soak in" the lessons. If you go straight to yang, not only will you learn poor technique, but your chances of injury while training will also be much higher.
- When an opponent strikes, you can receive his attack using yin, going with the flow of his motion. You may also defend against it using yang, attacking your opponent's limb as he strikes. A third option is to use a combination of yin and yang, where you receive the attack by flowing with it and then redirect the energy to counterattack.
- When you're using your hand to meet an attack, if your fingers face forward, it is considered yin. If your fingers face up, it's Yang. When your fingers are up, the hard, bony part of your hand is exposed, but when your fingers are forward it's not.

Related Chapters:

- Weight Distribution Drill
- Bombs
- Attack
- Stepping

PART I
HAND TO HAND COMBAT

STEPPING

Spring Semi-Forward Stepping

Spring semi-forward stepping is used to close distance.

In this movement, your back heel is up. This turns your calf muscle into a double spring—one behind your knee and one at your heel. Releasing these springs propels your whole body forward.

Take a small step forward with your lead foot and move your rear foot into the original position of your lead. Your stance should never be too exaggerated.

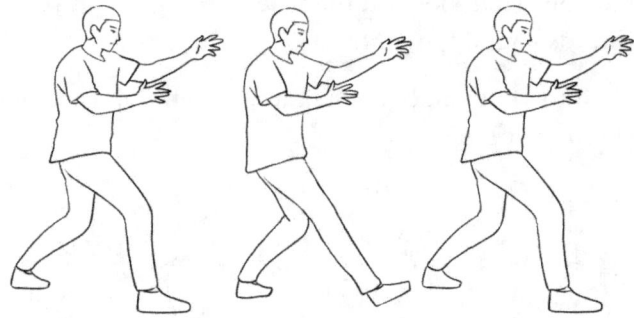

Keep most of your weight on your rear leg. The heel of your front foot should land first, followed by the toes of both feet. This will keep you well-grounded and ready for the next move.

When using the spring semi-forward step, you'll most likely be attacking, which means your attacking arm (usually your lead) will be at 160°, but never more.

Remember that 120° is the strongest angle for defense, and 160° is the best for offense. Never go outside of these angles.

Angulated Stepping

With this method of stepping, you close in on your opponent by going around him/her first. This allows you to:

1. Maneuver around any linear attacks.
2. Collect bodyweight to put more power behind your strike by grounding yourself.

To practice angulated stepping, start in a neutral position. Step towards your opponent, but at an angle. Always point your extremities towards your opponent—it will focus your power.

Change the direction of your toes to face your opponent. Put all your weight onto your lead foot and then step through with your rear leg, directly towards your opponent.

You'll "fall" into your opponent's space, which will put more bodyweight behind your blow.

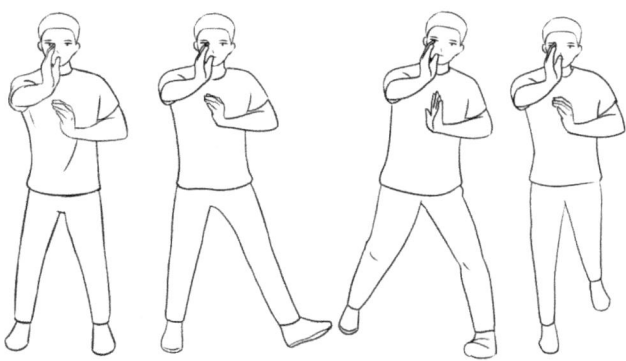

WEIGHT DISTRIBUTION DRILL

This drill trains your body to put weight behind your strikes. Start in a neutral stance, with your left hand up in a guard position.

Shift your weight onto your right leg as you turn your body to the right. Your left arm should come down as your waist moves, following the movement of your waist naturally manner. That is, your arm should move because of your waist motion.

Bring yourself back to a neutral position. Mimic defense with your left hand, using a 120° angle. Continue to turn to your left. Follow the movement of your waist with your right arm for a big hit.

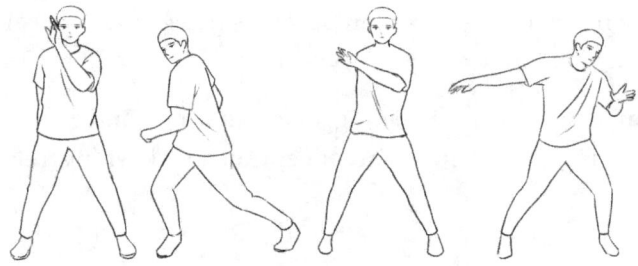

As you drop your weight onto your left leg, hook your right arm in to hit your opponent. Repeat the action from left to right, and so on.

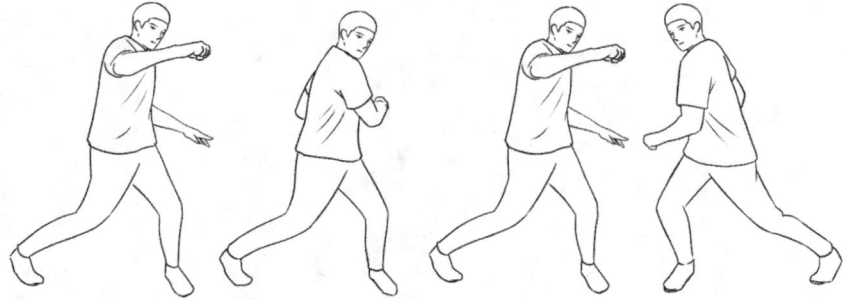

The above demonstrates big circular hitting, but the drill can also be applied to linear strikes.

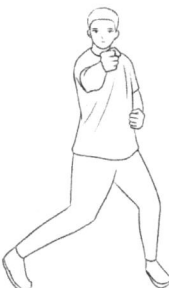

Whichever leg you're placing your weight on can be considered your brake. It grounds you. If you don't do this, you'll lose balance. At the end of the hit, that same leg then becomes the spring to accelerate the circular movement.

Once you're used to the feeling of grounding (and you can do it without losing your balance), concentrate on keeping relaxed and flowing.

BOMBS

Bombs are your first line of defense and offense. There are four of them.

Defensive Bomb

The defensive bomb is used for short-range defense. This move is used when you've been caught off-guard, so it's likely your hands will be down at the time. It's a "panic" move.

As soon as you notice the incoming attack, condense yourself down and in. Lower your weight to set a spring. This compression will also ground you, making you more stable. Explode out at your opponent. Put your head back and bring your lead knee up to face him/her. The motion should continue with you bringing your hands out into the ideal defensive angle of 120°.

In this move, your knee is weaponized. It can be used as usual or in a bomb-kick, crushing your opponent's leg (aim for his/her knee). Once you land, you "go to work" on your opponent with entries and follow-ups.

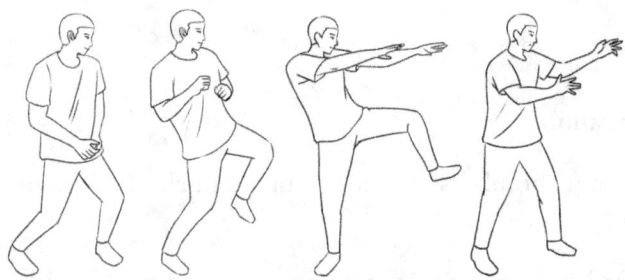

Bomb-Kick

The bomb-kick can be used with any of the bomb techniques. Its power is created by gravity and the "spring" in your leg muscles. You don't put any effort trying to kick through your target. Instead, position your knee as a defensive-aggressive weapon and then release the spring.

When you raise your leg in any of the bombs, ensure your knee comes up pointing towards your opponent. If it's to the side it can be easily pushed away.

Have your foot close to your bum. This "spring-loads" your leg. When you're ready, release the spring so your knee's angle is at 160°. Keep the 160° strong and then allow your body weight to push your foot through your opponent's leg. His/her knee is an ideal target.

A simple exercise you can do is to hold your leg in the "loaded" position and then let it "fire." The aim is to get a feel for stopping at the ideal 160° angle.

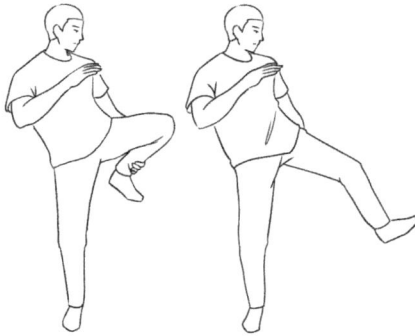

Hammer Bomb

The hammer bomb is a short-range attack. It is dynamic and explosive.

Bring your knee up facing your opponent and attack with your lead hand, using a hammer fist in the over-and-down waterfall action. This allows your arm to come over your opponent's limbs and onto his/her head and/or arms.

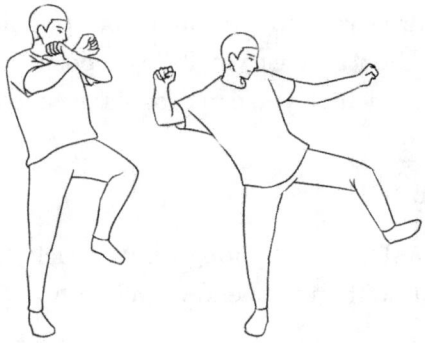

Pendulum Bomb

The pendulum bomb is a long-range attack. It's used when you decide to take someone on before they are close enough to become an immediate threat. Like a pendulum (hence the name) you rock your body back and forth.

First, present your opponent with a long-range weapon (your lead hand) as a feint. You want your opponent to think your hand is your attack, and perhaps even go for your head as a target.

Extend your rear limbs behind you to allow for more reach. As your opponent comes in, draw yourself back in and shift your weight to your rear foot.

Bring your lead knee up and weaponize it into a kick/stomp to your opponent's knee. Guard your head with your rear hand, although it (your head) will most likely be well out of range.

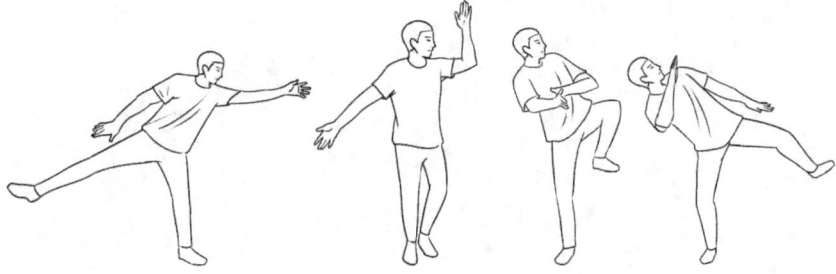

"Fall" forward to drive your foot through your opponent's knee. If you miss your target, then at least you'll be in position to take up your fighting stance, from which you can progress into more attacks.

Cross-Step Bomb

The cross-step bomb is a really long-range attack. It will cover about two feet more ground than the pendulum bomb.

Starting in a right lead stance, bring your left leg forward to cross behind your right. Your left foot should be angled to your rear. Put your weight on your left foot and bring your right knee up facing your opponent.

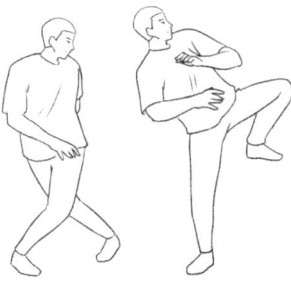

Extend your right foot to the optimal 160°. Fall into it, preferably with your foot crushing through your opponent's knee.

Take up your fighting stance and attack if needed.

Related Chapters:

- Attack

BOUNCING KICKS

Groin Kick

After you do a bomb, with or without the follow-through bomb-kick, instead of grounding your lead foot you can bounce it back up for a kick into your opponent's groin.

Do your bomb and then allow your lead foot to fall to the ground, but keep your weight on your rear leg. Bounce your foot back up into your opponent's groin.

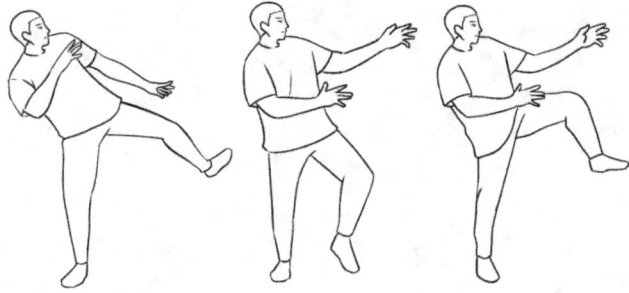

To practice this action, it may help to pretend your knee is like a basketball or yoyo.

Donkey Kick

It may be that you land behind your opponent after your bomb, or that someone approaches you from behind. In this case, you can use a donkey kick.

The same bouncing movement is used, but it's your heel that meets the target.

A variation of the donkey kick is to bring your foot straight up your back into your opponent's jaw. This can be useful if someone puts pressure on you from behind and you're forced to lean forward.

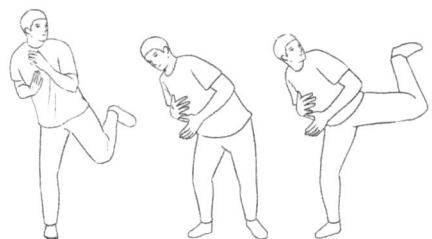

Turning Arm Strike

Another useful strike when someone forces you to lean forward is the turning arm strike.

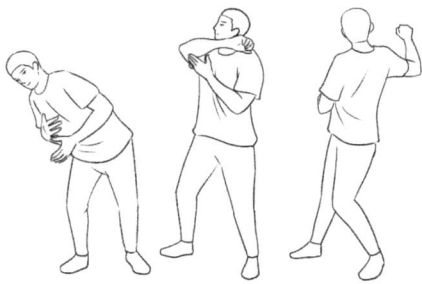

The striking point could be your elbow, forearm, hammer fist, etc.

ENTRIES

An entry technique is used to break through your opponent's initial guard. All the entry techniques described will take you up to the checkmate position.

The following picture illustrates the checkmate position. The main thing is that your arm should be on the outside of your opponent's guard.

Ideally, your arm will be tight against your opponent's. It's also preferable for you to use your non-striking hand to secure your opponent's arm—by grabbing his/her wrist, for example.

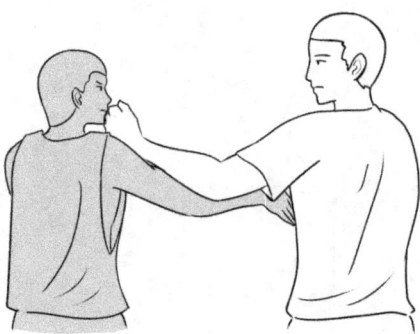

When adopting the checkmate position you may feel more comfortable stepping in, or perhaps stepping through (changing your lead).

The demonstrations show the entry using two hands. They can also be done one-handed. This is something you should experiment with during training.

All entries can be done with an almost simultaneous low kick, which will help confuse your opponent.

Techniques for getting from the entry to the checkmate position are not set in stone. A variety of ways have been demonstrated; these can be mixed and matched to get something that works best for you in a given situation. You should experiment with different starting positions so you can become aware of which entries work best for you in which circumstances.

Related Chapters:

- Stepping

SLAP ENTRIES

Slap entries are ideal to use when your opponent's guard is held out more than 160°, but they can also be used when your opponent's guard is within the power angles (120° to 160°). The basis of the slap entry is to knock your opponent's hand horizontally to clear a path for your attack. Often, the initial slap is a distraction technique. It's subtle, but helps to confuse your opponent.

Outside Parry Entry

Step in and use your lead hand to lightly tap and bounce off your opponent's extended arm at his/her wrist. Almost simultaneously, follow your lead hand with your rear to guide your opponent's arm to the outside so you command the centerline.

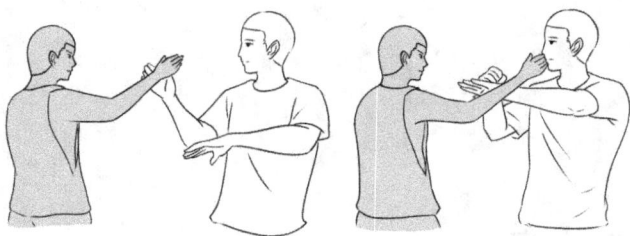

Strike your opponent with your lead as soon as your opponent's centerline is cleared. Next, cross your lead hand over to keep your opponent's lead under control while you strike with your rear.

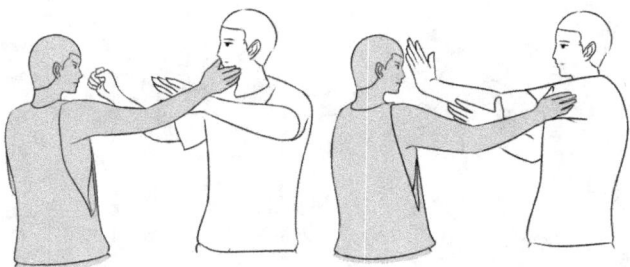

Use your right hand to guide your opponent's lead arm across his/her body. Strike your opponent's ribs. Notice the pointed knuckle fist in the image below, which is used to dig in between the ribs. A normal fist will also suffice.

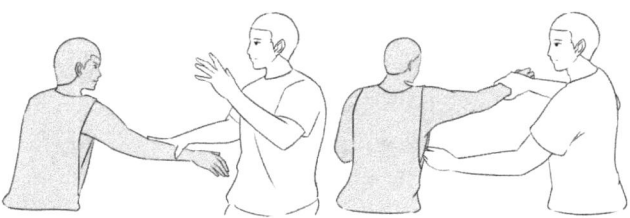

Without letting go of your opponent's wrist, adopt the checkmate position.

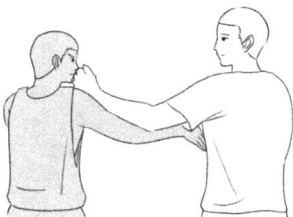

Inside Parry Entry

Use your lead hand to tap and bounce off your opponent's lead. Almost simultaneously, use your rear hand to slap your opponent's hand back to the inside of his/her body. Strike with your lead.

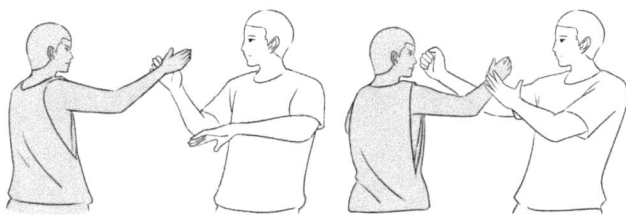

Bring your lead hand straight back and collect your opponent's lead hand on the way as you adopt the checkmate position.

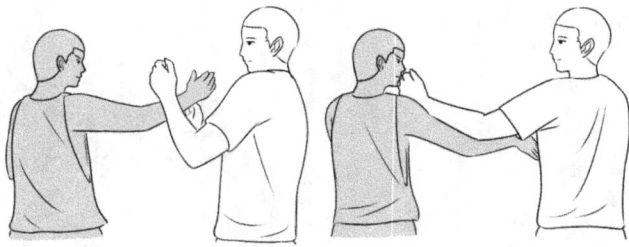

Flick Entry

With your lead hand, slap through your opponent's lower arm and bring it to your centerline.

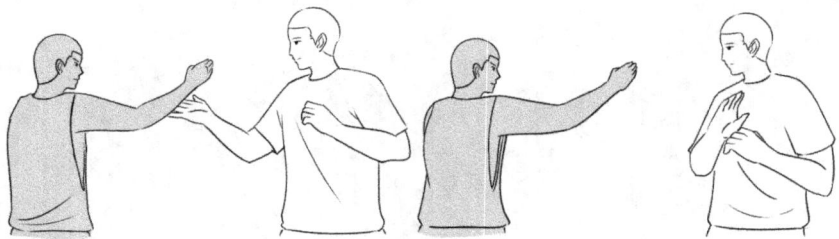

As you step forward, press you rear hand against your opponent's lead arm, just enough to clear the centerline so your lead can come through. Bring your lead hand straight back and collect your opponent's lead hand as you adopt the checkmate position.

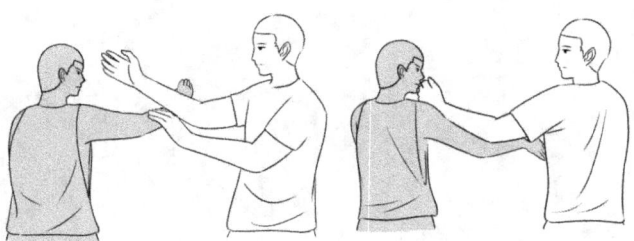

Hammer Entry

With your lead hand slap through your opponent's lower arm and bring it to your rear shoulder.

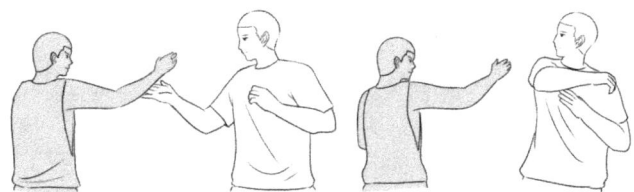

Crash down on your opponent's lead arm with your elbow as your hammer-fist strikes his/her face. Continue moving your lead hand along its path and collect your opponent's lead arm as you move into the checkmate position.

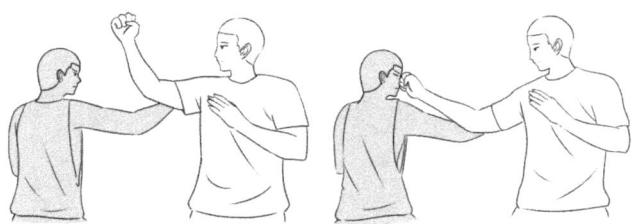

Step Entry

Take a step forward so that you switch your lead side as you close distance with your opponent. As you step forward use your rear hand (which will become the lead) to tap your opponent's lead from the outside, and then bounce off it.

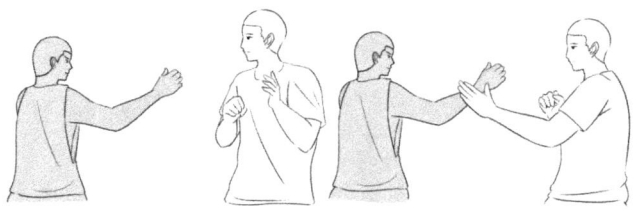

Almost instantaneously, use your other hand (your new rear) to take control of your opponent's lead as you adopt the checkmate position.

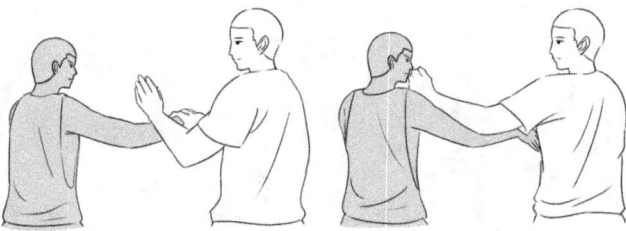

Elbow Entry

Your opponent may strike at you with his/her lead. Cover it with an inside parry. This is more of a backup action, and may not even connect.

As you do the parry, bring your lead elbow up on a vertical plane so that it deflects your opponent's arm to the outside of your body.

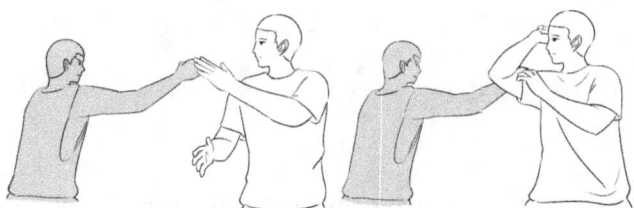

Come down on your opponent's lead with your lead. Do it hard, to hurt his/her arm. Use your rear hand to take control of his/her arm while striking with your lead.

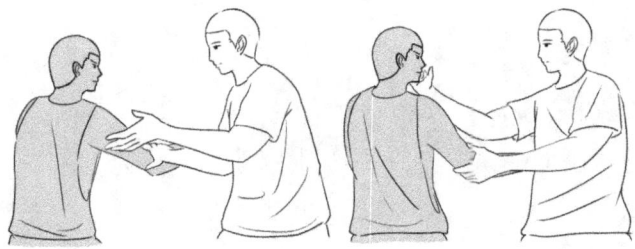

Take control of your opponent's lead with your lead and attack his/her ribs with your rear. Adopt the checkmate position.

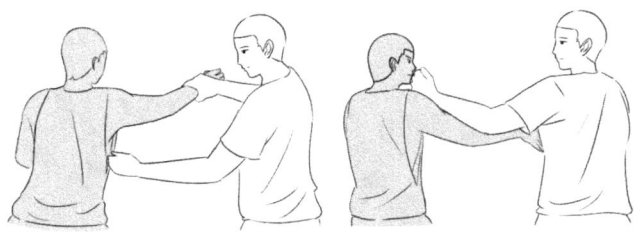

Alternatively, after step two (bringing your elbow up), you can drive your elbow forward into your opponent.

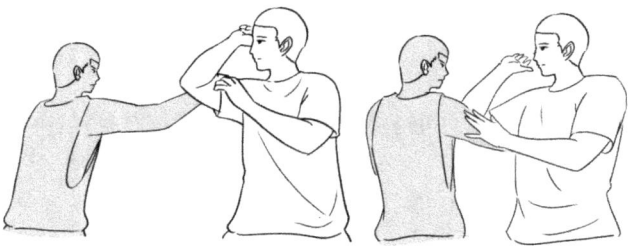

Hook Entry

The hook entry is a big strike entry that uses the hooking strike, as demonstrated in the weight distribution drill.

From the start position, let your lead drop and use your rear to guard your opponent's lead.

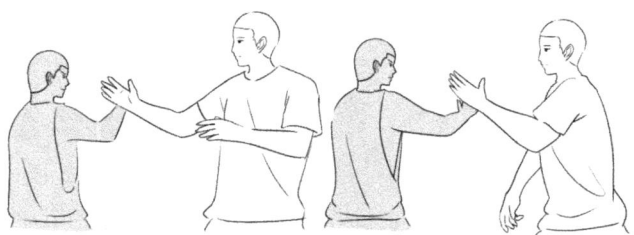

Move your opponent's lead down as you strike through him/her with your lead.

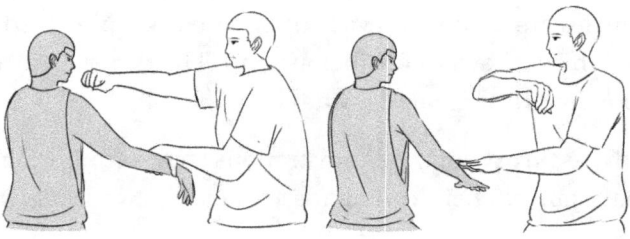

After doing the hook entry, you'll most likely go straight into the hand formula as opposed to checkmate.

Related Chapters:

- Weight Distribution Drill
- Hand Formula
- Attack

THRUST ENTRIES

Thrust entries are used when your opponent is keeping his/her guard too close to his/her own body (below 120°). The thrust entry collapses your opponent's lead hand in towards him/her.

Most of these thrust entry demonstrations start with both fighters in a right lead stance. Their lead hands are held out wrist-on-wrist.

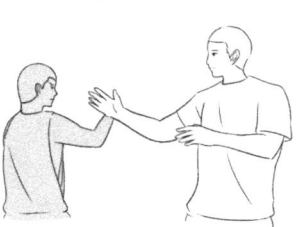

Push Entry

As you step forward, use your rear arm to apply pressure on your opponent's lead arm to clear the centerline. At the same time, strike with your lead.

The best place to apply the pressure is on the forearm, closer to your opponent's elbow. If you're too close to the wrist, your opponent may be able to strike you with his/her elbow.

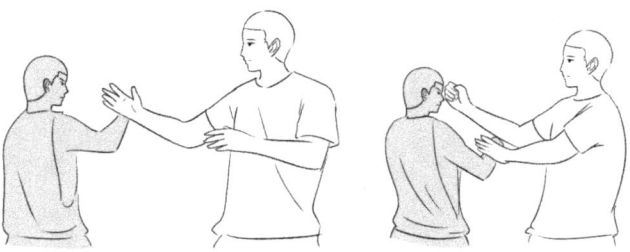

Bring your lead hand straight back and collect your opponent's lead hand as you adopt the checkmate position.

Neck Attack Entry

With the neck attack entry, you drive your lead forearm into your opponent's neck.

As you move forward, use your rear hand to clear the centerline by applying pressure to your opponent's lead arm. Target his/her upper arm/shoulder. Apply the pressure on a "rolling angle" across his/her body and slightly back towards yourself.

At the same time, attack your opponent's neck on an upward angle with your forearm. As your forearm comes into contact with your target, you can give it a little forward torque.

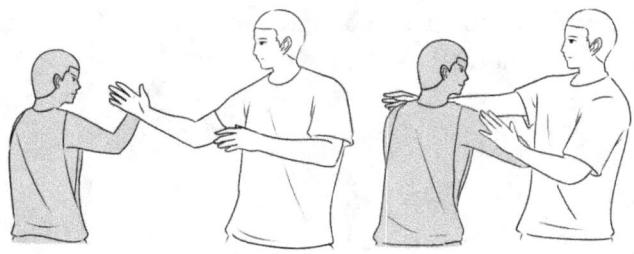

From there, move into the checkmate position.

For a less brutal strike, aim for the chest as opposed to the neck.

When you perform this move, it's important for you to stay grounded. Even when your opponent is slightly taller than you, it is possible.

Don't come up on your toes. Instead, ground your left side more and extend the right side your torso.

If needed you can double up on your attack. This may be useful if your first strike missed your target, and/or if your opponent is attempting to grab your arm.

Sink your weight and drop your arm. Sinking your weight resets your spring. Dropping your arm will clear (and hurt) your opponent's arms while creating space for you to repeat your attack.

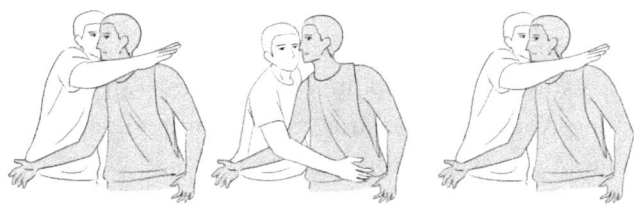

The Push-Neck Combination

The push-neck combination is the push entry immediately followed by the neck attack entry. It's a good demonstration of how entries can flow from one to another.

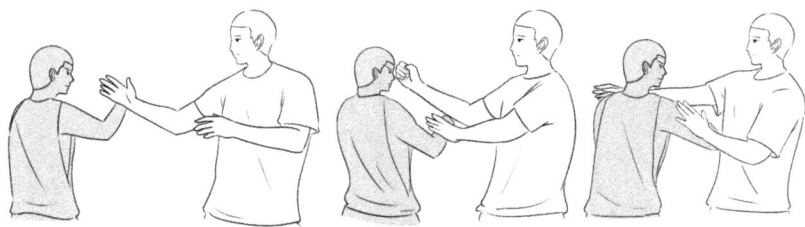

Related Chapters:

- Attack

CURVE ENTRIES

Curve entries go around your opponent's guard in some way. When making one, be careful not to open yourself up. Stick to his/her arm, or as close to him/her as you can.

Curve-In Entry

Curl your lead hand around your opponent's, towards the inside of his/her guard. Next, use your rear hand to quickly guard his/her lead as you strike with your lead.

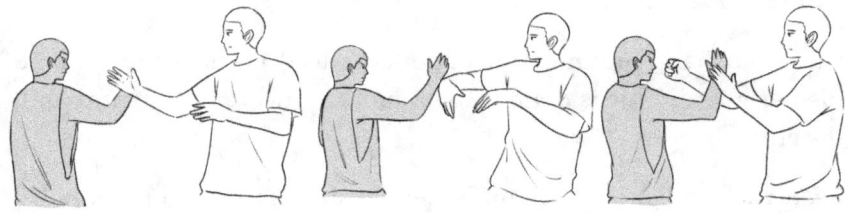

Collect your opponent's lead with your lead and strike with your rear to adopt the checkmate position.

Tap-Curve Entry

Move into the starting position with a slight tap to your opponent's hand and then quickly withdraw.

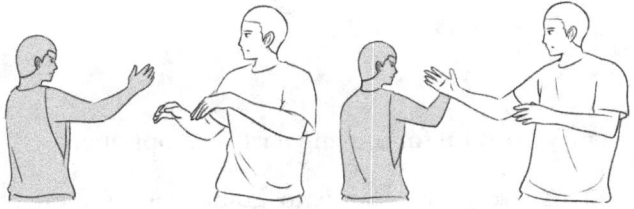

The act of tapping your opponent's hand from one side will cause him/her to resist. It is a feint.

Your opponent's opposing movement leaves his/her centerline open. Strike, and then adopt the checkmate position.

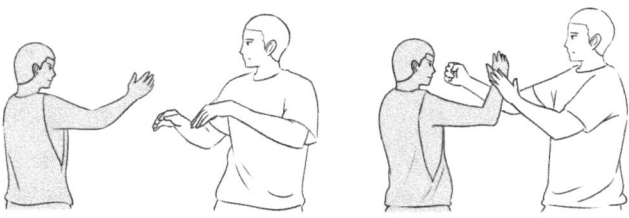

Curve-Under Entry

Curl your hand around your opponent's lead towards the inside of his/her guard. This is done using a more vertical movement than in the curve-in entry.

Lean back and strike from underneath using an upward motion. Use your rear hand to guard your opponent's lead. Adopt the checkmate position.

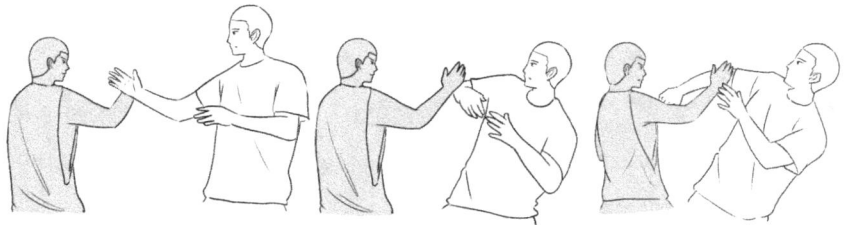

Groin Entry

The groin entry is useful for moving past your opponent.

Step in and use your rear hand to guide your opponent's elbow past you.

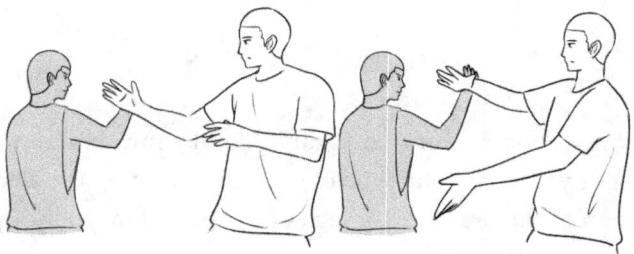

Curve your lead down to attack your opponent's groin.

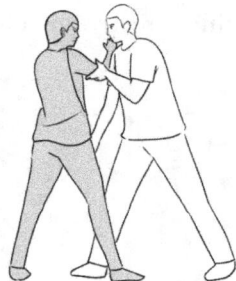

If you're not moving past your opponent, you can go into the checkmate position by bringing your rear hand up the outside of your opponent's guard and then using it to pull his/her lead towards you.

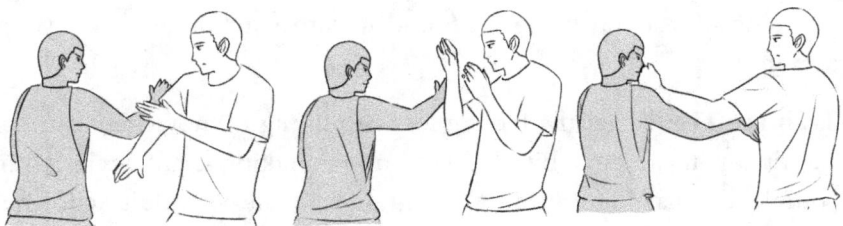

CONTACT ENTRIES

When using a contact entry, you grab hold of your opponent's limb to shift it out of your way. The type of contact entry you use depends on the direction of the pressure (or lack of it) applied by your opponent.

Grab Contact Entry

When your opponent applies forward pressure. flow with it by grabbing his/her arm and moving directly into checkmate.

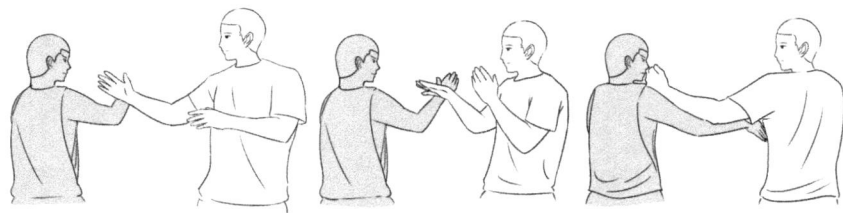

Hook Contact Entry

Use a big rear hooking strike while you pull your opponent in with your lead. Rotate your arm at the shoulder to gain tremendous momentum. As you bring it around toward your target, hook your arm in.

Training Tip: To get the feeling for the pulling-in movement during training, you can get a bit of a wind-up by making small circles with your lead wrist before doing the grab. Use the waterfall action to move over and grab your opponent's wrist.

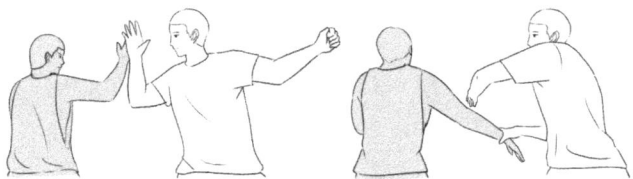

Bring your lead arm back to collect your opponent's arm, twisting him/her back in the opposite direction as you strike with a lead hook.

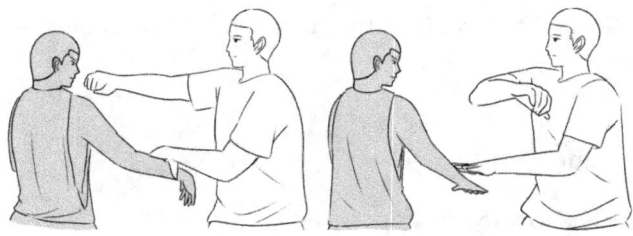

From this position, either continue with the hand formula or go into checkmate.

Push Contact Entry

Use this type of contact entry when your opponent is releasing pressure towards him/herself. Take advantage and pin his/her lead with yours as you strike, then adopt a variation of checkmate.

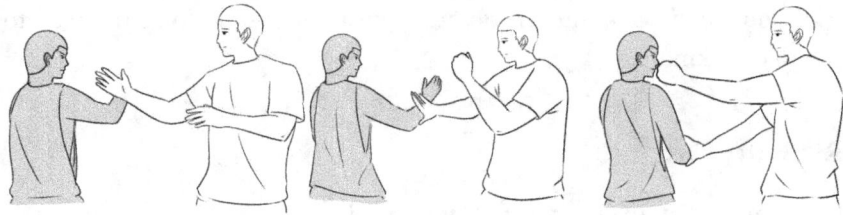

Related Chapters:

- Hand Formula

RIB ENTRIES

The main characteristic of a rib entry is that you attack your opponent's ribs.

Rib Entry One

Bring your lead over your opponent's.

At the same time, use your rear hand to guide your opponent's lead to the outside of your guard as you strike his/her ribs.

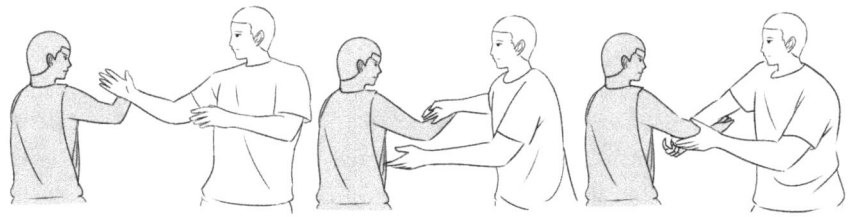

Pull your lead back and grab your opponent's lead along the way to adopt checkmate.

Rib Entry Two

Curl your wrist around your opponent's in the same manner as in the first curve entry.

Guard your opponent's lead with your rear as you strike his/her ribs.

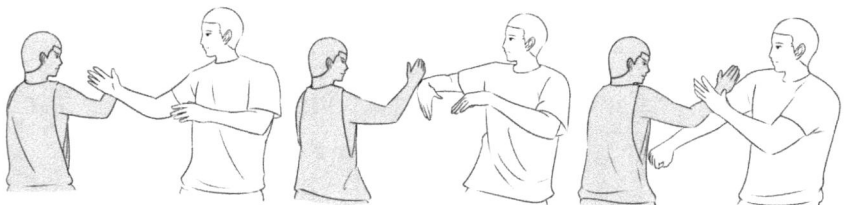

Rib Entry Three

Use your lead hand to guide your opponent's lead towards you.

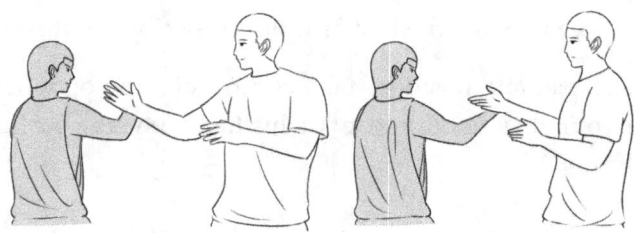

Once your opponent's lead has been extended far enough, use your rear hand to guard his/her lead from behind as you strike the ribs.

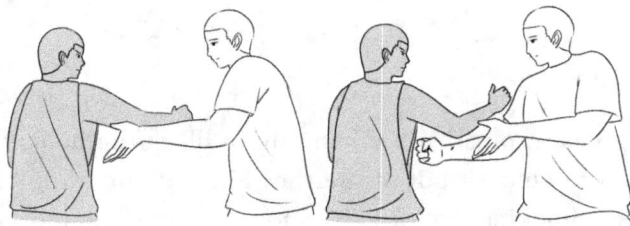

In variations two and three, adopt checkmate by bringing your rear hand up the outside of your opponent's guard and using it to pull his/her lead.

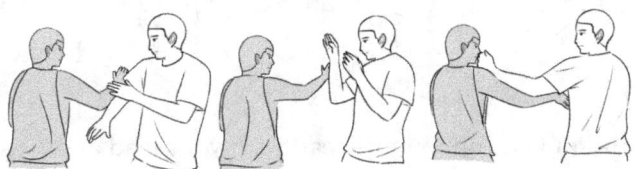

Related Chapters:

- Curve Entries

HAND FORMULA

Once you have completed your entry and achieved the checkmate position you can go into the hand formula described in this section.

From the checkmate position, take control of your opponent's lead arm with your rear hand and twist his/her body as you hook with your lead.

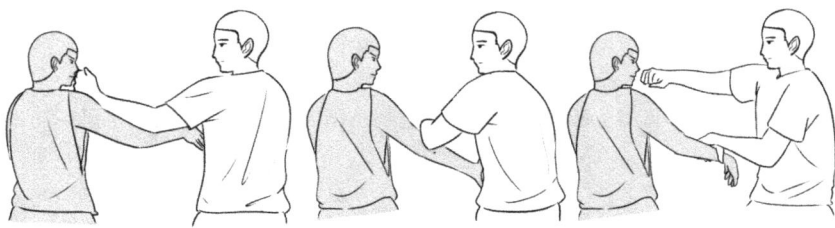

If your opponent puts his/her hand up to block the hook, curl your wrist down to guide it out of the way. Finish the curling circle and continue the hooking motion. This should be one fluid movement.

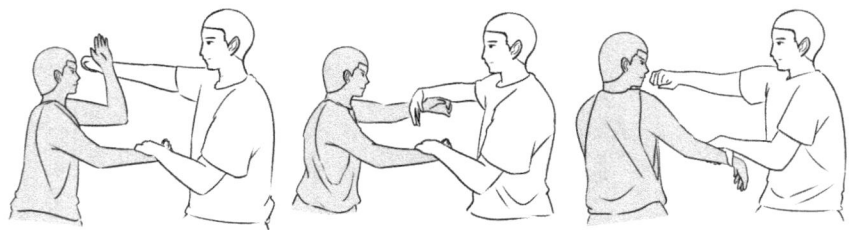

Take control of your opponent's lead with your lead and twist his/her body back the other way. Attack your opponent's ribs.

Use both your hands to jerk your opponent's lead arm down. Drop your weight into it to create a whiplash effect.

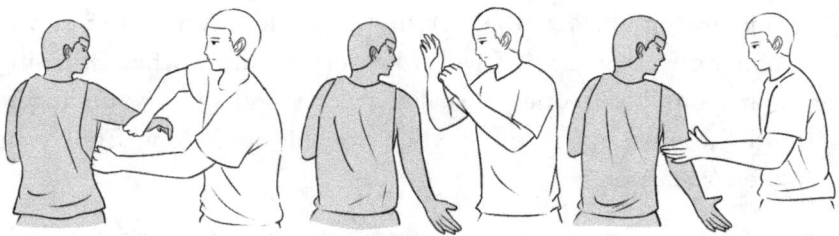

Immediately after pulling your opponent down, bring your lead hand back up to strike him/her underneath the jaw.

Pull your opponent's rear shoulder as you push on his/her lead upper arm to twist him/her back towards you.

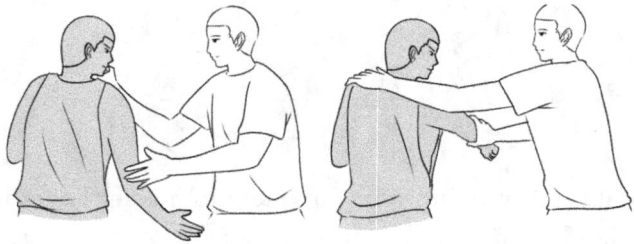

Bring your opponent to his/her knees by simultaneously applying pressure on his/her supra-scapular nerve and using the heel of your foot to push down and forward on the top of his/her calf, just below the knee. How exactly you do this will depend on your angle in relation to your opponent.

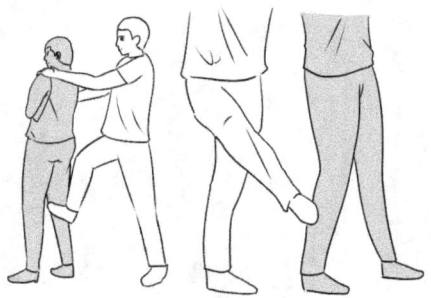

The picture on the left (below) shows the location of the supra-scapular nerve. You don't have to be very accurate when applying pressure point techniques. Just dig in, rub, and press your fingers around the area. You'll know when you hit something from your opponent's reaction.

Chop down on your opponent's supra-scapular nerve and then cup your hands and clap them on your opponent's ears. That is, press his/her head in between your hands.

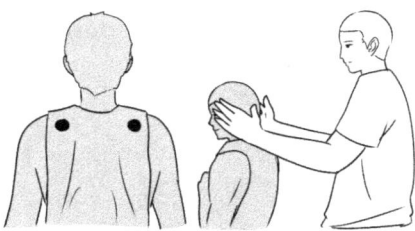

An alternative to bringing your opponent to his/her knees is to do a big hammer-fist strike over your opponent's shoulder. His/her solar plexus is the ideal target.

Apply a choke hold by circling your arms around your opponent's neck and then squeezing them together. Wrap your left arm around the front of your opponent's neck and grab your right elbow. With your right hand along the back of your opponent's neck, grab your left elbow.

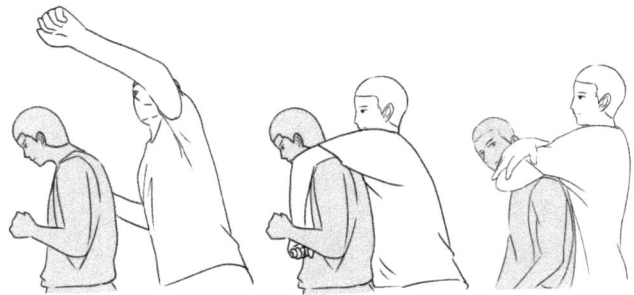

This choke could also be applied once your opponent is on his/her knees.

It's important to know that you don't have to get to checkmate before starting the formula, and in a real fight, you probably won't need to go through the whole formula. Often, just the entry will be enough to finish a fight.

Furthermore, you need not perform the parts of the formula in order. All the elements of Vortex Control Self-Defense, like any martial art, can (and should) be intertwined and used as appropriate for the circumstance and according do your opponent's reaction(s).

Here are just a few of the uncountable variations that you may choose to use:

After attacking the ribs, move directly into attacking your opponent's back.

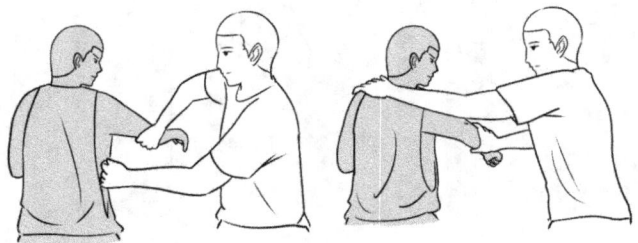

After the hammer entry, move directly into arm pulling.

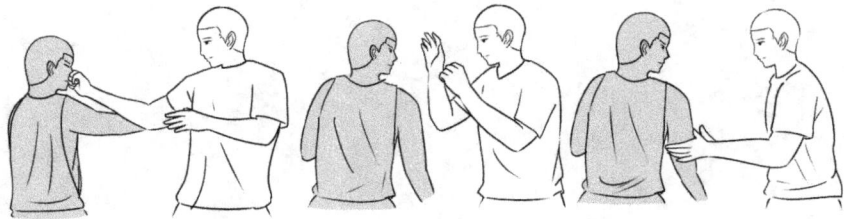

Move back into check-mate after attacking your opponent's ribs. You can repeat this move multiple times.

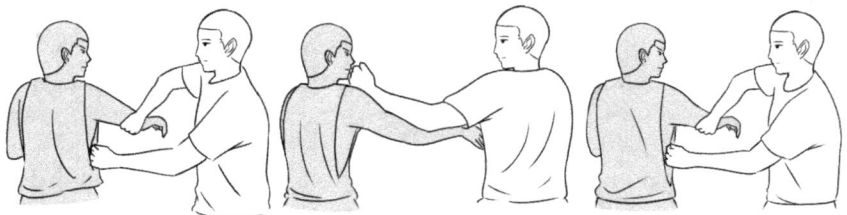

After the hook, move into an underarm pressure lock.

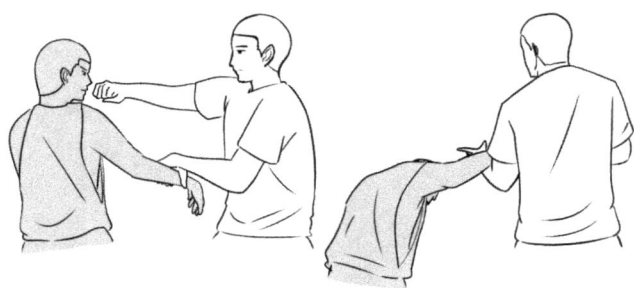

Related Chapters:

- Attack
- Lock Flow Drill

LOCK FLOW DRILL

The purpose of the lock-flow drill is to teach a wide variety of arm-locks. The term arm-lock encompasses the shoulder, wrist, fingers, etc.

In a self-defense situation, these locks can be used individually or in small combinations to serve your purpose.

Some reasons you may want to apply an arm lock are to:

- Gain pain compliance (to escort somebody out of a room, for example).
- Break an opponent's limb, which is likely to end the conflict.
- Disarm an armed assailant.

When practicing the following lock-flow drill, keep these points in mind:

- As you flow from lock to lock, always have at least one hand griping your opponent's limb. This helps to keep him/her from escaping.
- You can slide your hands along your opponent's limb while still keeping your grip. You'll get better at this with practice.
- Where possible, keep your elbows close to your body. This will enable you to best use your center of gravity to generate power.
- Jerking, vibrating, strikes, etc., can be used to soften your opponent up, making it easier to apply the locks effectively, and/or to increase the damage done. Some examples of these things are included in this chapter's demonstrations.

For ease of remembering and writing, the following locks have been given semi-descriptive, unofficial names.

Shoulder Lock

From the checkmate position, use your left hand to move your opponent's right hand down. At the same time, move your right hand towards your opponent's left shoulder.

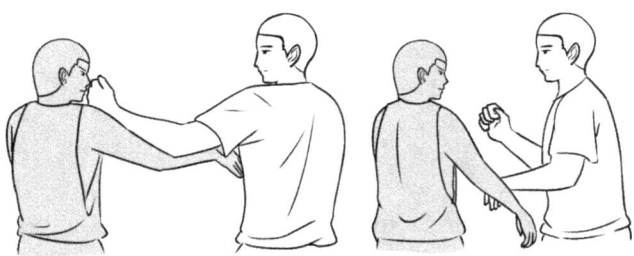

Move your left arm under your opponent's arm to his/her rear, so that the underside of your elbow, which is facing up, can hook onto his/her arm.

Bend your opponent forwards by applying pressure on his/her shoulder with your right hand.

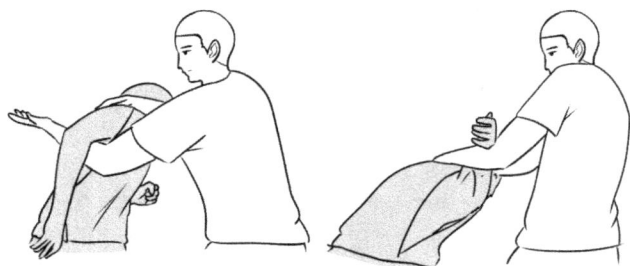

Here, the shoulder lock is shown from the opposite side, and aggression is added.

With the hand that isn't hooking your opponent's arm, strike his/her face on the way to grabbing his/her neck.

As you come back to grab your opponent's neck, do so forcefully, using a cupped hand.

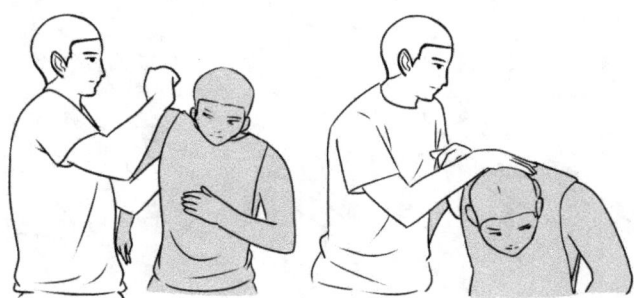

Follow up with another elbow to your opponent's head. You can repeat these two strikes, You can also knee him/her.

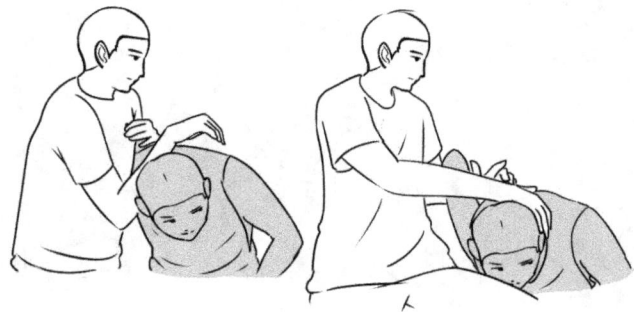

Wrist Twist

Slide your right hand down your opponent's arm to control his/her elbow. At the same time, slide your left hand down and grip at your opponent's wrist.

Your left hand should be on the inside of your opponent's guard, with your palm facing out.

Grip your opponent's wrist and then pull his/her arm across your centerline.

You can use your right hand to help with a push at your opponent's elbow, although this is usually not needed.

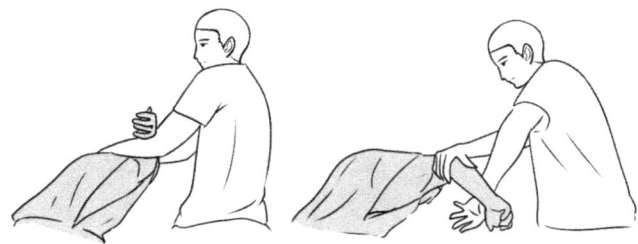

As you bring your opponent's arm across your centerline, continue to slide your right hand down his/her arm to meet your left hand at his/her wrist. Use both your hands to bring your opponent's hand up and then over to the outside of his/her guard. Use the waterfall principle.

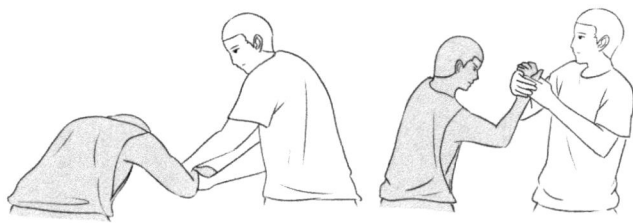

When the wrist twist is fully applied, it has the potential to damage the whole limb.

Wrist Twist Variation

Release the pressure and then apply a variation of the wrist twist by pushing your opponent's wrist down towards him/her.

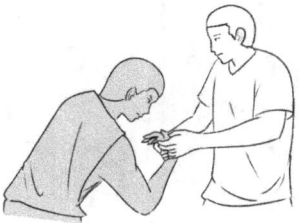

Wrist Lock

As you release the pressure from the wrist twist variation, grip your opponent's fingers with your right hand. Push your opponent's hand into his/her face.

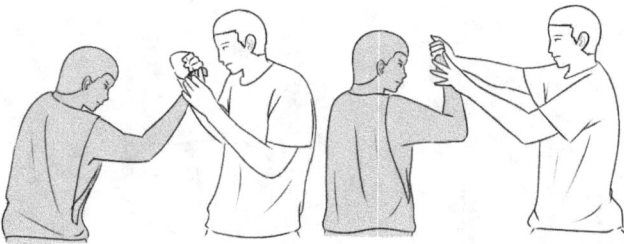

Move your left hand to your opponent's elbow. Push your opponent's elbow as you pull his/her fingers down and towards your centerline.

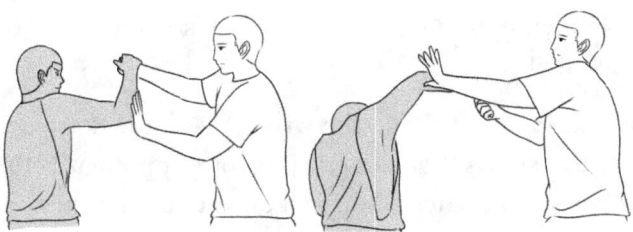

As your opponent's arm straightens, grab hold of his/her thumb with your left hand and then pull his/her hand towards your center. Lock your elbows close to your body and apply torque his/her hand, applying pressure (creating a vortex), to perform the wrist lock.

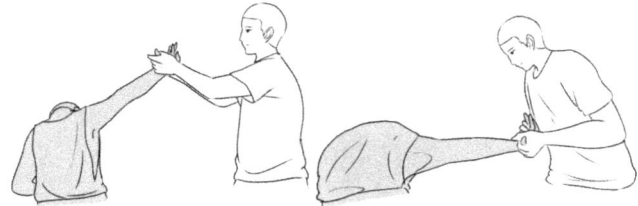

Wrist Pressure

Keep a good grip on your opponent's thumb with your left hand while sliding your right hand up to his/her elbow. Bend his/her arm down vertically at the elbow and use a circular motion to move it to the inside and up.

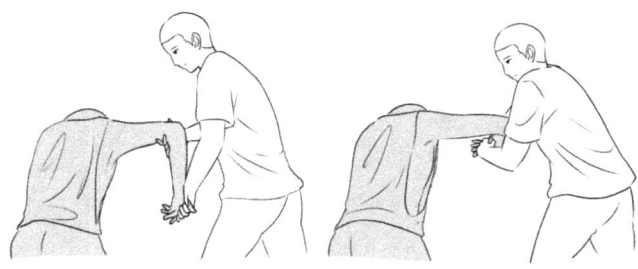

Use your right hand to help place your opponent's upper arm securely in the crook of your elbow. Apply pressure on his/her wrist with your left hand to cause pain and lock his/her arm in. You can use your right to strike.

The image on the right shows the wrist pressure lock from the opposite side. It also shows that you can put your opponent's elbow either on your bicep or your chest. Putting it on your chest is more secure.

Instead of striking, you can also use your spare hand to increase the pressure on your opponent's wrist.

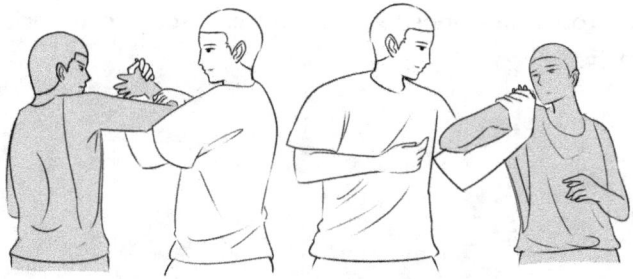

Overarm Pressure

Grip your opponent's wrist with your right hand and then curl your left arm underneath his/hers. At the same time, pull his/her arm straight with your right hand.

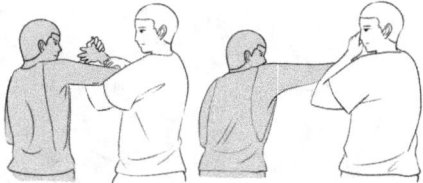

The end result will be that your opponent's arm is straight and his/her elbow faces up. Apply pressure on his/her elbow with your forearm.

As you apply pressure down with your left, pull up with your right. At the same time, use a waterfall motion by applying pressure with your forearm as you roll it over your opponent's elbow.

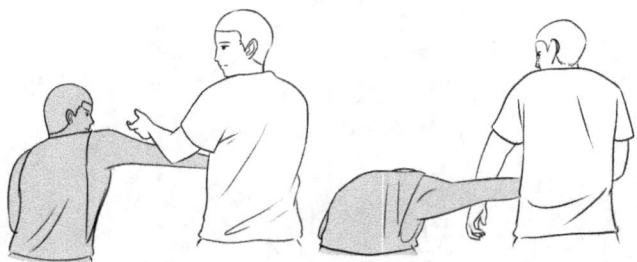

Here it is from the opposite side. You can see the waterfall action more clearly.

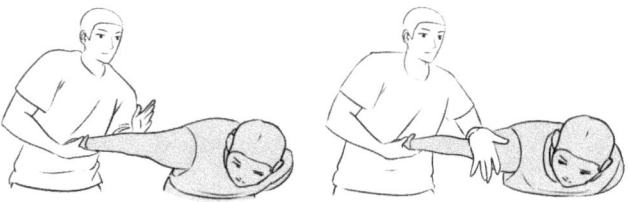

Underarm Pressure

Curl your left slightly toward yourself and then underneath your opponent's arm.

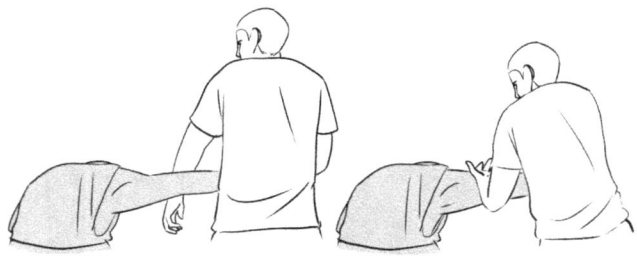

As you do this, your opponent's arm is rolled so that his/her elbow faces the ground.

You apply upward pressure on your opponent's elbow with your own elbow. Your left palm faces up. Apply downward pressure on his/her hand with your right hand.

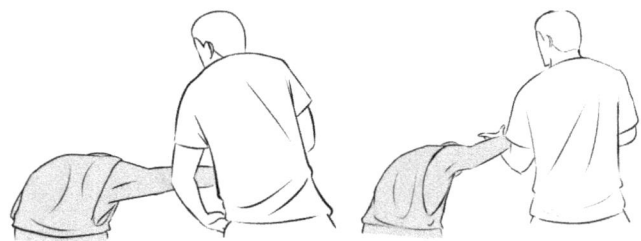

Here it is from the opposite side.

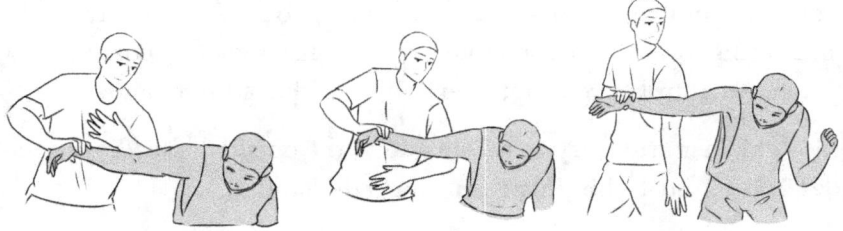

Bent Arm Lock

Return to the overarm pressure lock and then, without letting go of your right hand, bend your opponent's arm towards him/her and grab your right wrist with your left hand. Strike your opponent with your right elbow.

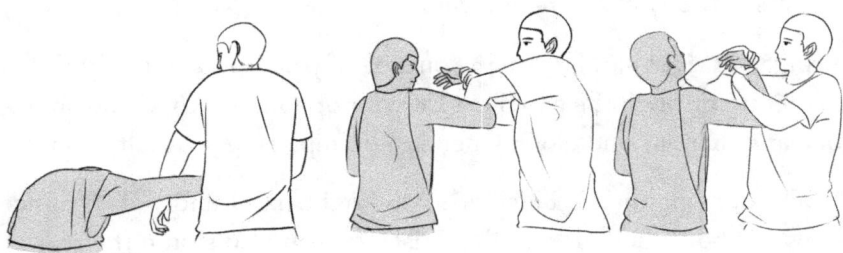

Here it is from the opposite side. Once your arm is on top, you can strike at your opponent's eyes before bending his/her arm.

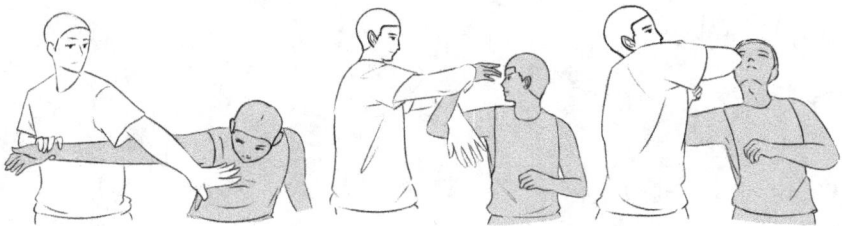

One-Handed Bent Arm Lock

Let go of your right wrist and grab your opponent's fingers from the side facing towards you, so that your palm faces your opponent. Now you have control of your opponent's limb with your left hand.

Move his/her arm away from you and to the outside of his/her shoulder. You can strike him/her with your right hand.

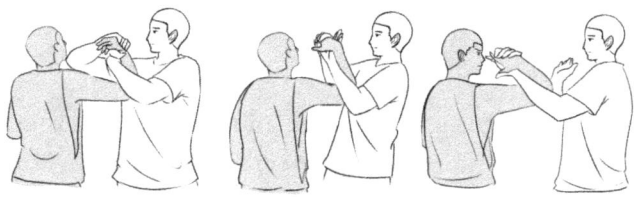

Reverse One-Handed Bent Arm Lock

Bring your right hand up on the outside of your opponent's right arm. Pass it up through the gap between your opponent's wrist and shoulder, and then take hold of his/her fingers, replacing your left hand.

Grab your opponent's hair with your right hand and pull him/her down by both the hair and the wrist. You can also stomp the rear of your opponent's knee.

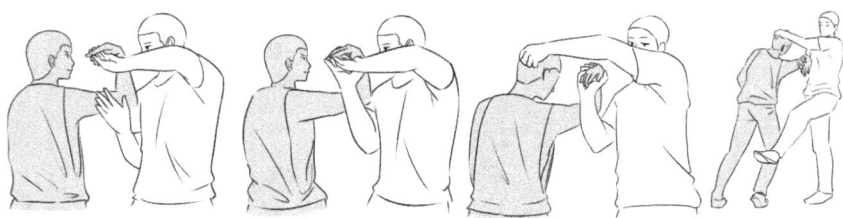

Crooked Elbow Lock

Swing your left arm between your opponent's wrist and shoulder until the crook of your elbow is on the crook of his/her elbow, with your palm facing up. As you do this, release your right hand and catch his/her wrist under your armpit. Apply upward pressure with your left arm.

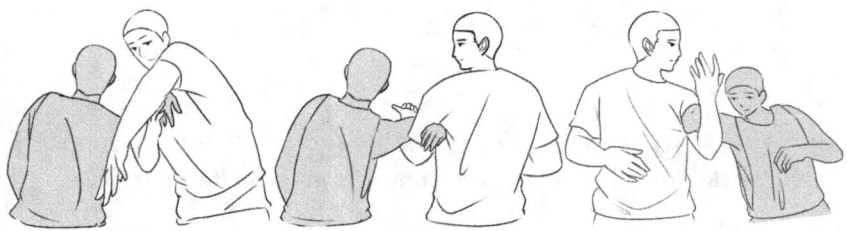

Over-Shoulder Arm Bar

Reach over with your right arm, grab your opponent's left wrist, and pull it towards you. Pass it across your opponent's body, in between his/her body and your left hand.

Place your right hand on the back of your opponent's left shoulder and your left hand on his/her lower left arm, twisting his/her body towards your left shoulder.

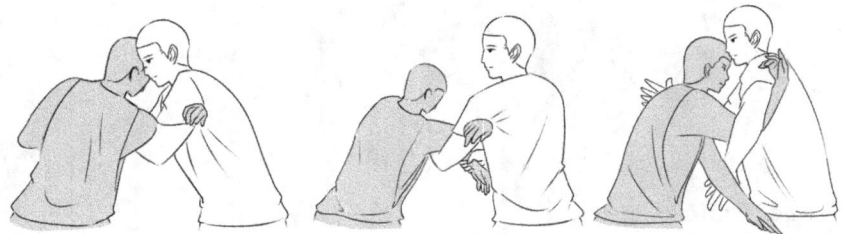

Drop your left arm and use it to attack your opponent's neck. The twist-and-strike action should occur very quickly so you can use the momentum it creates to put more force behind the strike.

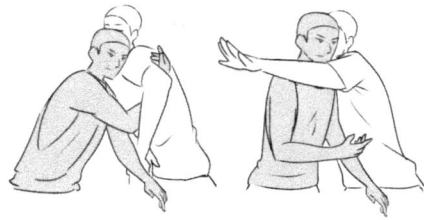

Turn your body so that you're facing the same way as your opponent. At the same time, drop both your hands to grab his/her left hand.

When you drop your hands, be sure to keep your opponent's arm between them. Grab your opponent's wrist with your left hand and take hold of his/her fingers with your right.

Continue to turn your body to the left as you straighten your opponent's arm over your shoulder. His/her elbow should sit on your shoulder, with the underside of the elbow facing up. Pull down on your opponent's wrist to apply pressure.

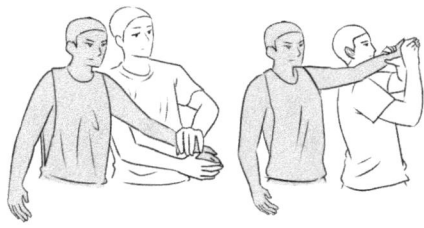

Finger Control

Use your right hand to grab your opponent's ring and pinky fingers. Bend those two fingers down back towards him/her. As you do so, bring his/her lower arm down so that it's aligned along the top of yours. Keep your left hand on his/her wrist.

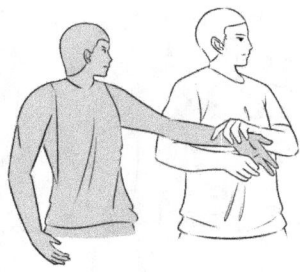

Begin to spin your opponent, so that you swap sides. Do so initially by bending his/her fingers back as you apply pressure on his/her left arm with your right arm.

Keep your opponent's hand near your waist for better leverage on his/her fingers. Pain compliance will keep him/her spinning once your lower arms lose contact.

Finger Lock

Towards the end of the spin, as your opponent is still spinning, use your left hand to grab his/her index and middle fingers.

The third image below shows the finger grab from the opposite side.

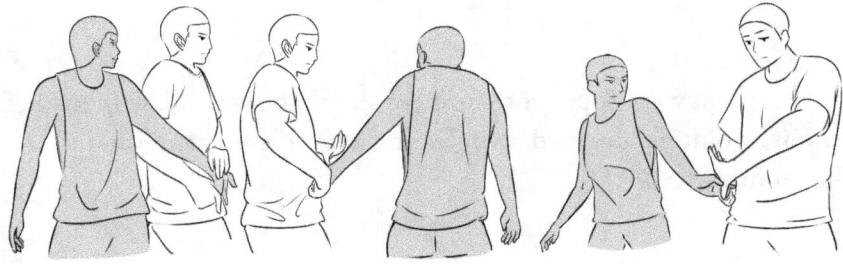

Keeping your opponent's arm straight, bring his/her hand up with his/her bent fingers pointing up. Jerk your opponent's hand down towards you.

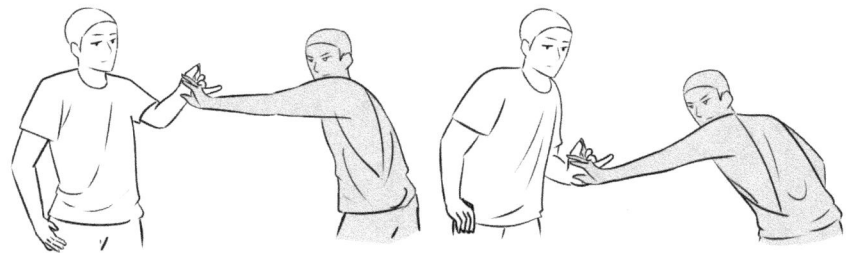

Forearm Torque

Bring your right arm, with your palm facing up, under your opponent's left arm. Place the crook of your elbow just above your opponent's elbow.

Grab your opponent's right wrist with your right hand. Pull his/her hand down by the wrist while applying pressure on his/her elbow with your right arm.

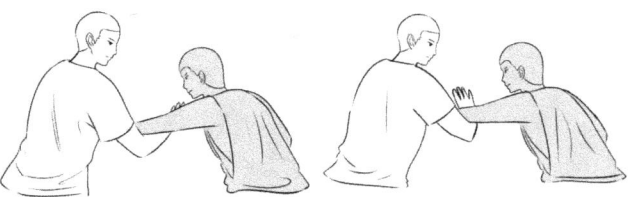

At this point your opponent's forearm should be vertical, with his/her elbow pointing upward, while his/her upper arm should be horizontal.

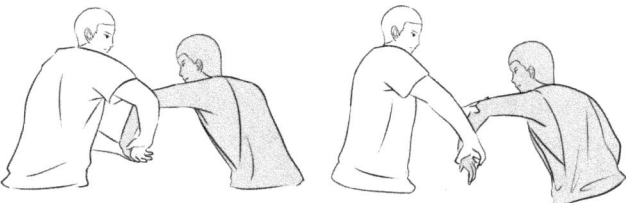

This completes the basic lock-flow drill.

Lock-Flow Drill Alternatives

Now a few (of countless) alternative movements are shown to demonstrate how the drill can be altered depending on the situation at hand.

Wrist-Twist Alternative

This demonstrates how you can go back to the formula from the lock-flow drill. It also shows how you can flow from the rib entry to an upward chin strike as opposed to going to checkmate and then the formula.

At the end of the wrist twist, release the pressure on your opponent's wrist and strike him/her in the ribs, as you would in the rib entry.

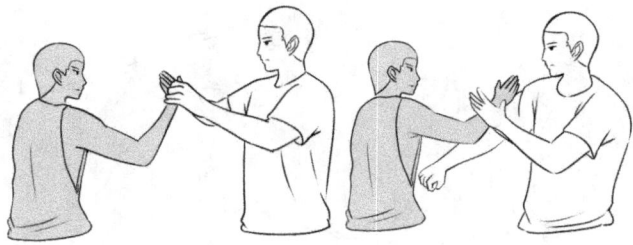

Continue with the rib entry as normal by bringing your hand up to the outside of your opponent's guard.

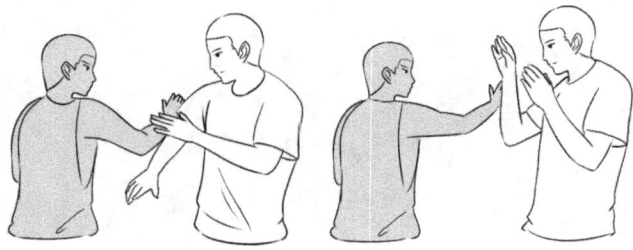

Instead of going into checkmate, you can go straight into the arm pull, and follow it with an upward palm heel to your opponent's jaw.

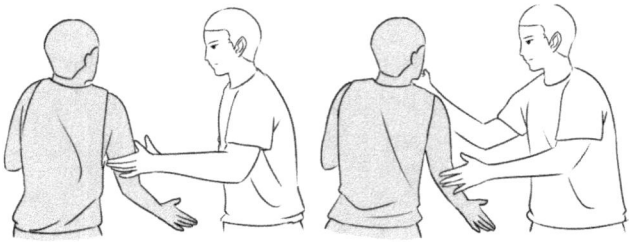

Crooked Elbow Lock to Figure-4 Arm-bar

After you release the pressure from the crooked elbow lock, it's possible for your opponent to swing at you. Use a variation of the elbow entry to block the attack. For example, raise your right elbow.

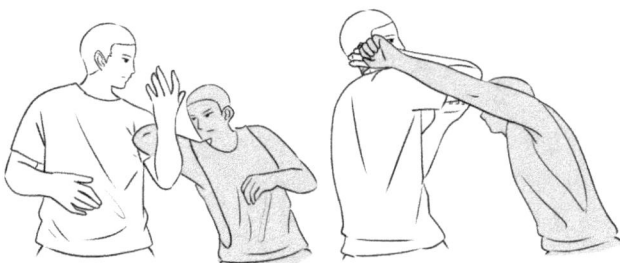

Capture your opponent's arm by circling your right arm over his/her left arm. At the same time place your left hand on your opponent's right shoulder.

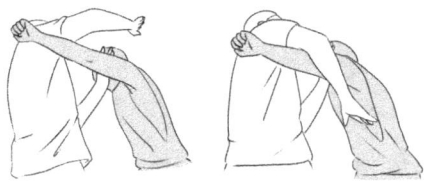

Grab your left forearm with your right hand. Your opponent's straight arm should be in the crook of your right elbow. Apply the figure-4 arm-bar by pushing down on your opponent's shoulder while applying upward pressure on his/her elbow. As you release the lock, strike your opponent's solar plexus with your right hand.

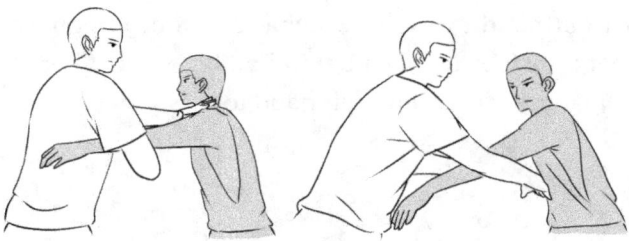

Slide your left hand down your opponent's left arm and grab hold of his/her wrist. As you do this, give him/her a right hook to the jaw. Continue into the over-shoulder arm bar.

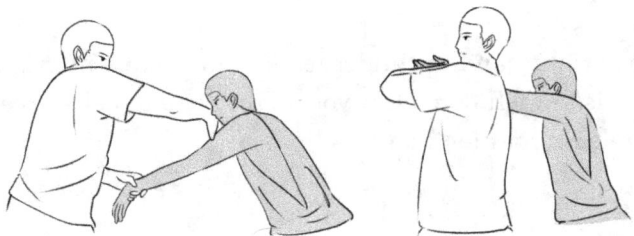

Alternative Ending

This demonstration gives a different ending to the lock flow drill. It starts from the finger lock. Bring your opponent's fingers up to the right side of your chest. With your left hand deliver an uppercut underneath your opponent's left arm to his/her jaw.

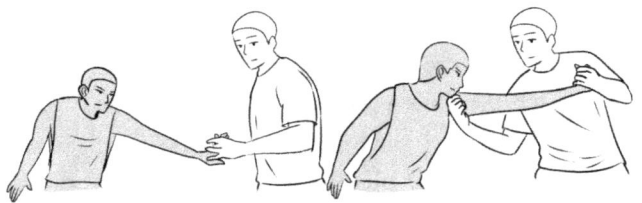

Use your right hand to control the back of your opponent's head so you can bend his/her left arm behind and down his/her back. You'll need to adjust the grip of your left hand to do so.

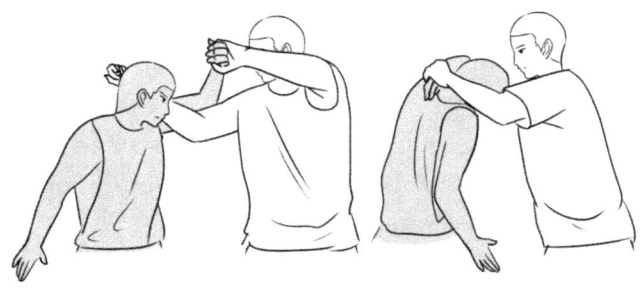

Bring your right hand up underneath your opponent's right armpit and grab his/her left hand. Use your right hand to help force it down. You can release your left hand.

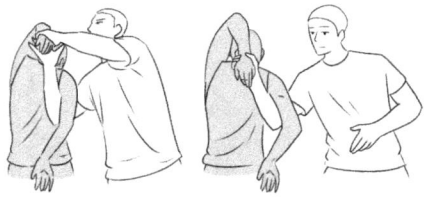

Related Chapters:

- Rib Entries

PART II
KNIFE DEFENSE

ATTACK

In the demonstrations in this book, the attacker will always hold the knife in his right hand. When the description refers to a left attack, it means one in which the strike comes in on an angle from the attacker's left. The knife is still held in his right hand.

Note: The method of attack used in this book is intended to help you practice defense. For more effective knife attack methods, please refer to the bonus chapters.

Straight Thrust

A straight thrust is when an attacker strikes into your torso from waist height. It's always done using a forward grip.

Downward Stab

As its name suggests, the downward stab is an attack that comes in on a downward motion. It's always done using a reverse grip.

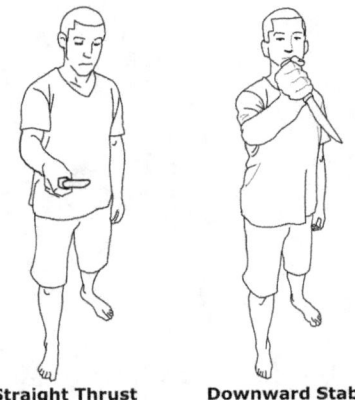

Straight Thrust   **Downward Stab**

Related Chapters:

- Bonus Chapters

DEFENSE

Every defense begins with the block/grab technique. This allows you to have two hands on your attacker's one, and is important because it gives you better control of his knife-wielding hand.

Unfortunately, using the block/grab technique ties up both your hands. This makes you vulnerable to being hit by your attacker's other hand, especially if you're slow to apply a disarm.

However, being hit is better than being stabbed, which (arguably) makes the block/grab a safer technique to use than others.

Unless otherwise stated, your grabbing hand is closer to your opponent's hand than your blocking hand is. You block on your opponent's lower forearm, but grab at his wrist.

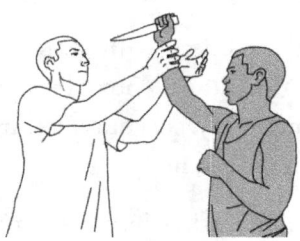

Blocks

There are two main types of blocks for knife defense: the chop and Bong Sau. How these blocks are applied depends on the situation, as well as on what works best for you.

To do the chop, use your forearm to chop down on your attacker's arm. Do it hard and aim for his upper forearm, since there is a cluster of nerves there. Often, this blow on its own will be enough to cause your attacker to drop his knife.

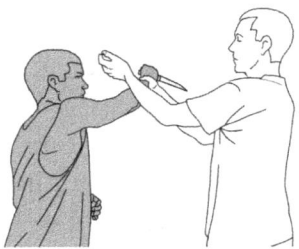

Bong Sau is taken from Wing Chun, but its application is modified depending on the situation. The images offer the best interpretation.

What follows is another excerpt *Basic Wing Chun Training* by Sam Fury.

Bong Sau (wing arm) is a defensive technique unique to Wing Chun. It's used to divert a punch by creating an angle of deflection.

Begin in the half squat position, with your hands up. In one movement, turn your hand down and your elbow up. As you do so, turn your waist and tilt your body so your feet are in a fighting stance. Your waist should do the work, not your arm.

Keep your arm in line. You other hand is a guard hand in case your opponent's strike passes through. This is Bong Sau.

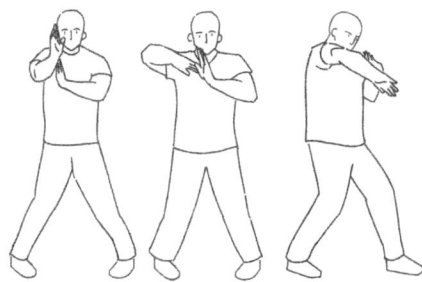

Turn slightly back and bring your hand back to the center.

Switch hand positions so your other hand becomes your lead. Shift your weight to match your new position and then do Bong Sau on your other side.

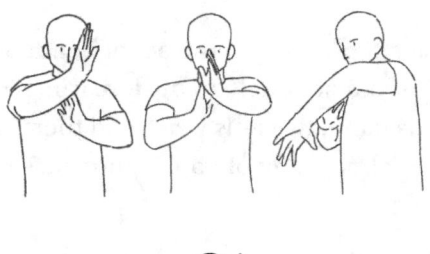

Grips

There are two types of grips.

An underhand grip is when your palm faces up or to the outside of your opponent's guard.

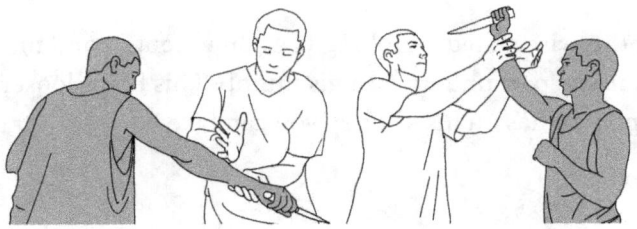

An overhand grip is when your palm faces down or to the inside of your opponent's guard.

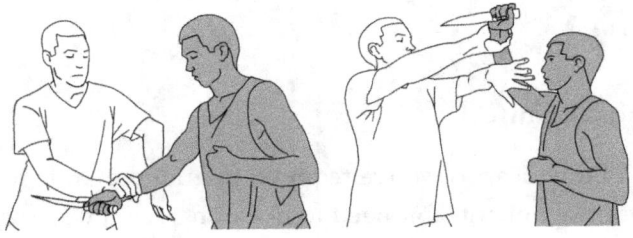

Making a Tap

In many of the disarms, once you've applied the block/grab technique, the next step is to "make a tap."

The term "making a tap" refers to the act of bending your opponent's wrist so his hand is at a 90° angle to his forearm. Doing this makes it easier to control his hand, twist his wrist, and therefore disarm him. A tap can be made at almost any of your opponent's joints. This makes it easier to apply locks.

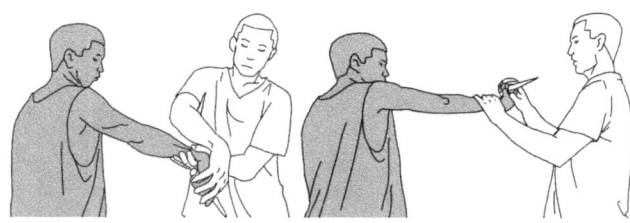

Grabbing Your Opponent's Hand

Unless otherwise stated, grabbing your opponent's hand means grabbing the fleshy part underneath his thumb. This helps loosen the grip your opponent has on his knife so you can take it.

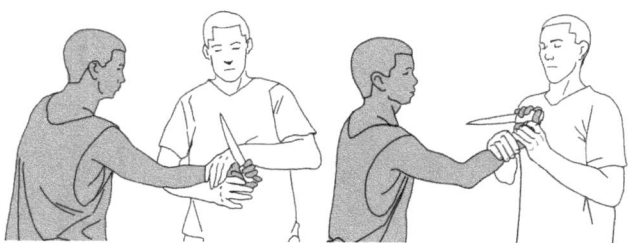

Grabbing the Knife

In many of the disarms, you're required to grab the knife in order to disarm your opponent. You need to do so in such a way that you do not cut yourself.

Grabbing the handle is the best way, but this won't be possible most of the time because your opponent will be gripping the handle. The next best option is to grab the blade from the blunt side. This assumes it is a single-edged knife.

The last option is to grip the blade between your fingertips and your palm in such a way that the sharp edge does not touch you.

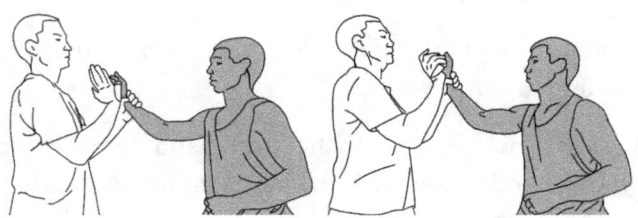

Aim to grab as much of the handle as possible when doing this, to minimize injury.

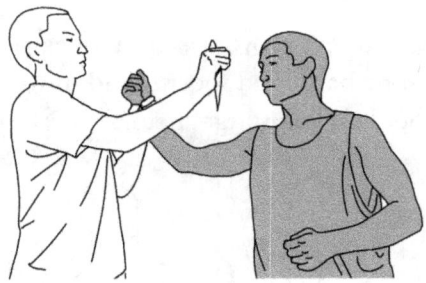

Taking the Knife

In most cases, you'll pull the knife towards your opponent's thumb and pry it out of his hand. This will take advantage of the weakest point in his grip.

KNIFE STEPPING DRILLS

These simple drills ingrain the foot to step in with in your muscle memory.

Knife Attack Stepping Drill

In a knife attack, step in using the foot on the same side as your knife strike is coming from.

The same side is not necessarily the same hand. In other words, just because you're holding the knife in your right hand doesn't mean the knife is coming in from the right-hand side.

Stand with your feet shoulder-width apart. This is the neutral position. Hold the knife in your right hand near your right shoulder, with a reverse grip.

At the same time, step in with your right foot as you stab down with your right hand. Your hand and foot should move at the same time, but your hand should hit your target before your foot lands.

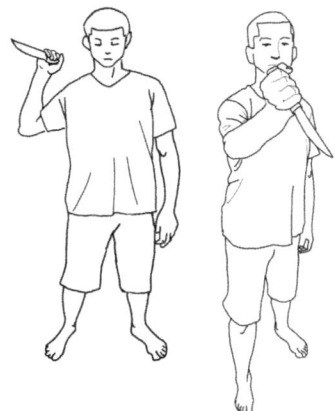

Step back to your original position with your right foot. As you do, bring your right hand to your left shoulder.

Step in with your left foot as you stab down from your left shoulder with your right hand.

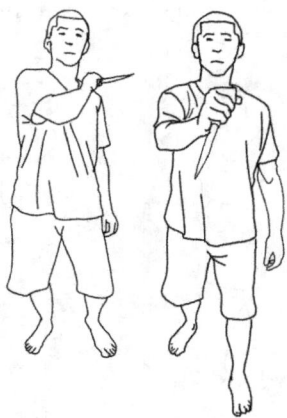

Return to the starting position and repeat the previous movements for a few minutes. When you're ready, change to a forward grip and hold the knife in your right hand near your right hip. Place your feet in the neutral position.

Step forward with your right leg and stab at the same time.

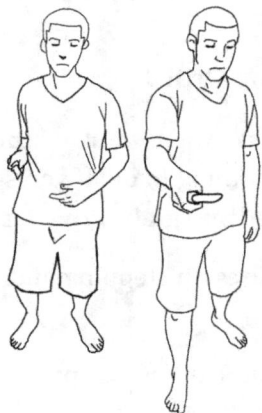

Step back into the neutral position as you bring your right hand back to the left side of your body. As you pull your hand back, rotate it so your palm faces up. This allows you to keep your knife pointed towards your opponent.

Step forward with your left foot and stab at the same time.

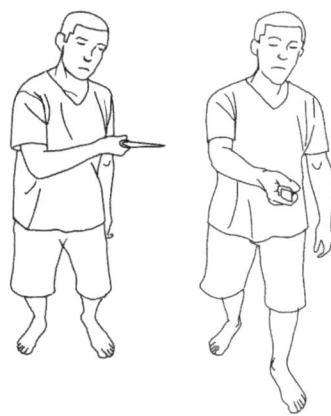

Return to your starting position and repeat the drill for a few minutes.

You can also go straight from the first part of the drill into the second. That is, you can do a right downward stab, left downward stab, right straight thrust, and left straight thrust.

Knife Defense Stepping Drill

In knife defense, it's best to step in using the foot that's opposite the side the knife attack is coming in on. If you step in with your left foot, block with your left hand and grab with your right, and vice versa.

The following drill focuses on stepping and blocking using the same hand.

Start in the neutral position, hands empty.

Step forward with your right foot and bring your right hand down to chop your imaginary opponent's forearm using a similar action as in the downward stab.

Use power angles (between 120° and 160°) at your elbow and wrist, with your fingers pointing towards your opponent.

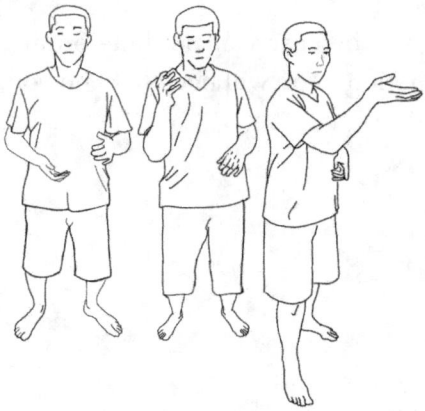

Return to the neutral position and then do the movement using your left side.

Next, do the same thing using Bong Sau.

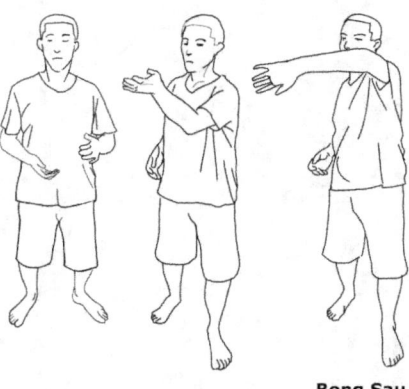

Bong Sau

The attack and defense drills can be practiced at the same time if you have a partner. One person attacks and the other defends.

The explanations of the drills shown above use simple angles and minimal body movement. This is for ease of explanation, but it's also a good place to start in practice.

In reality, attack and defense can be done on any angle, including curved hooking motions. You will need to bend your body depending on the situation.

Related Chapters:

- Attack
- Defense

GROUP A

Group A knife-defense techniques have the aim of taking the knife away from your attacker, and they all follow a similar pattern:

1. Block/grab.
2. Hand/thumb grab.
3. Create a "tap" (or twist the limb).
4. Disarm your opponent.

A1

Your opponent attacks with a right downward stab. Step in and block with your right using Bong Sau. Almost simultaneously, grab your opponent's wrist using an underhand grip.

Without losing contact with your opponent's arm, use your right hand to grab his right hand. Grab as much of his thumb as much as you can.

As you do this, turn your body so you are facing to your left.

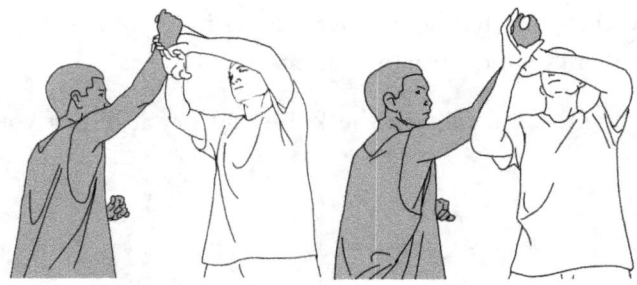

Bring your opponent's arm hard against your torso, at about the height of your solar plexus. If you haven't already, get a good grip on his thumb with your right hand.

Use your left hand to pry the knife out of your opponent's grip.

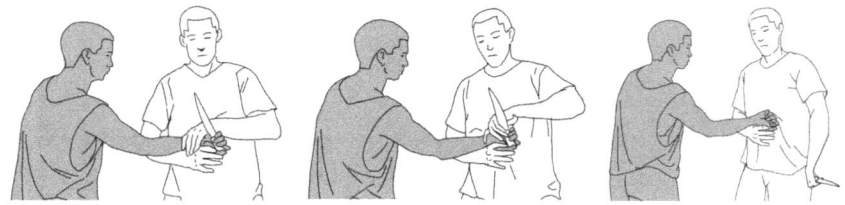

A2

Your opponent attacks with a left downward stab. Block with your left, using a chop. Grab your opponent's wrist with your right, using an underhand grip.

Use your left hand to grab your opponent's hand. Grab as much of his thumb as you can.

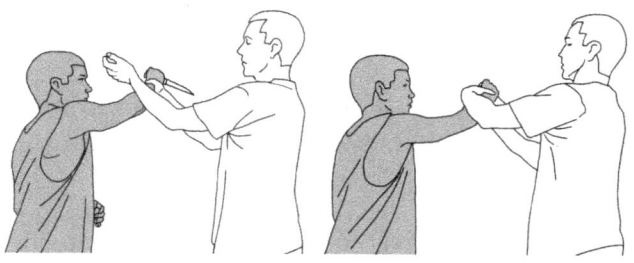

As you turn to your left, draw your elbows in to your body and bring your opponent's hand close to your chest.

Use your right hand to grab the knife and pry it out of your opponent's hand.

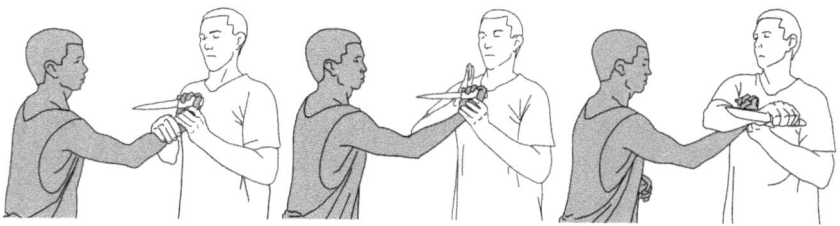

A3

Your opponent attacks with a right straight thrust. Defend with a right chop and left underhand grab. Use your left hand to grab your opponent's hand and bend his wrist down.

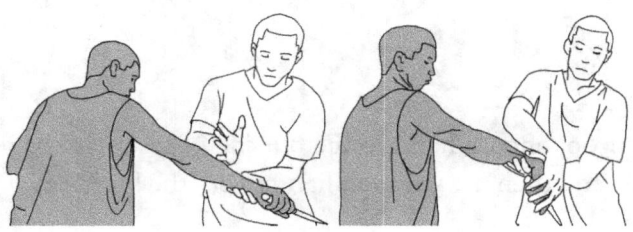

Without letting go of your hands, turn to your right so you're facing your opponent. This untwists you and leaves your opponent's elbow and hand facing up. Pry the knife toward your opponent to disarm him.

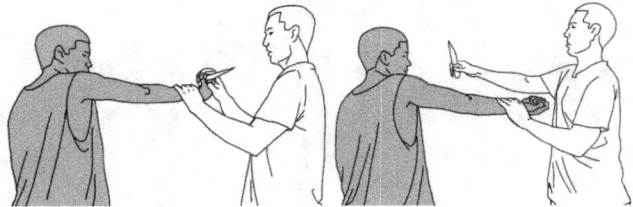

A4

Your opponent attacks with a left straight thrust. Chop block with your left and use an underhand grip with your right.

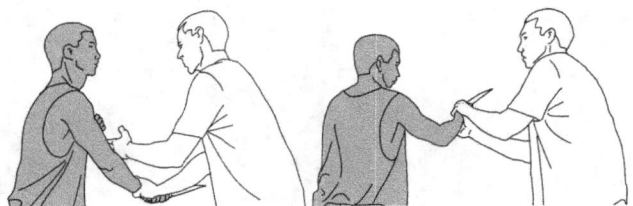

Use your left hand to grab your opponent's thumb, and then bring his hand up vertically.

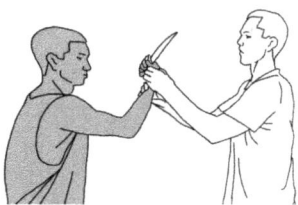

Bend your opponent's hand to the outside of his guard to perform a wrist lock, and then use your left hand to pry the knife out.

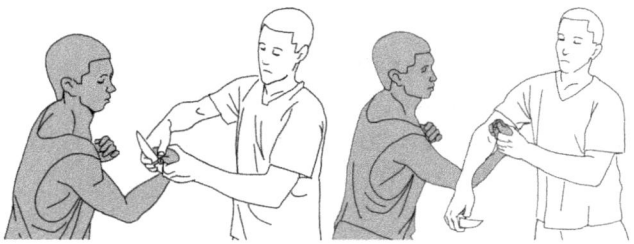

Related Chapters:

- Defense

GROUP B

Group B techniques are used to inflict pain on your opponent.

The pattern is:

1. Block/grab.
2. Trap your opponent's hand.
3. Induce pain.
4. Disarm your opponent.

B1

Your opponent attacks with a right downward stab. Defend with a right Bong Sau and left underhand grab.

Without losing contact with your opponent's arm, use your right hand to grab his right hand so that he cannot let go of the knife.

As you do this, turn your body so you are facing to your left.

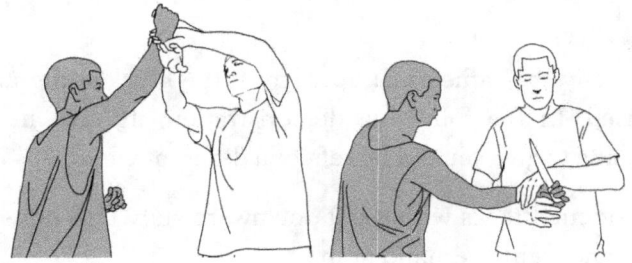

Bring your opponent's arm hard against your torso at about the height of your solar plexus.

Lean forward slightly to apply pressure and cause pain.

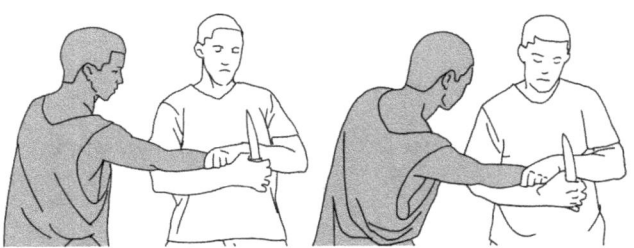

Release the pressure and then turn to face your opponent, while keeping hold of his arm.

Make the same downward motion to produce pain again, and then take the knife from your opponent.

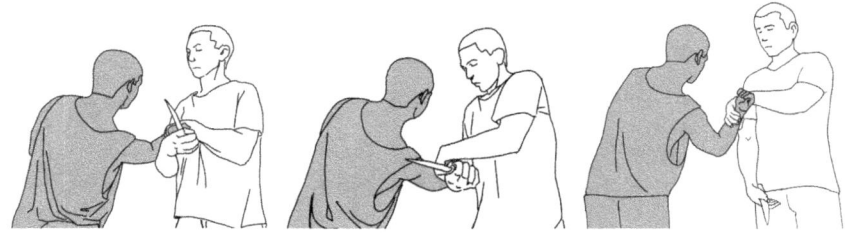

B2

B2 is basically the same as B1 apart from the block-and-grab combination used. In the following demonstration, it's shown from the opposite side to give you the benefit of a different view.

Your opponent attacks with a left downward stab. Defend with a left Bong Sau and right overhand grab.

Without losing contact with your opponent's arm, use your left hand to grab his right hand. Grab your opponent's hand so that he cannot let go of the knife. As you do this, turn your body so you're facing to your right.

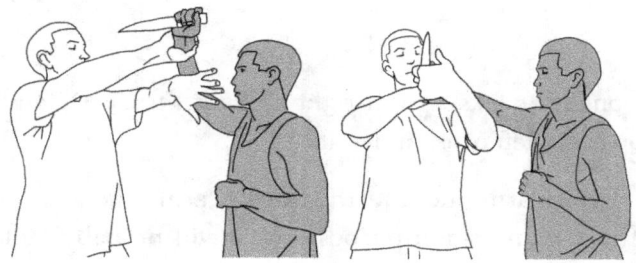

Bring your opponent's arm hard against your torso at about the height of your solar plexus.

Lean forward slightly to apply pressure and cause pain.

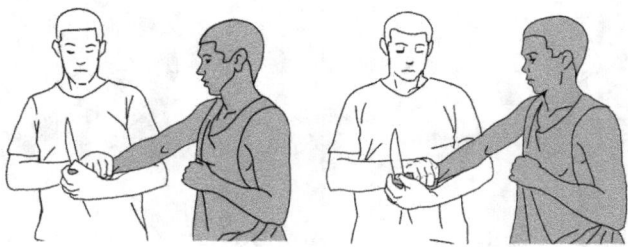

Release the pressure and then turn to face your opponent, while keeping hold of his arm.

Make the same downward motion to produce pain again, and then take the knife from your opponent.

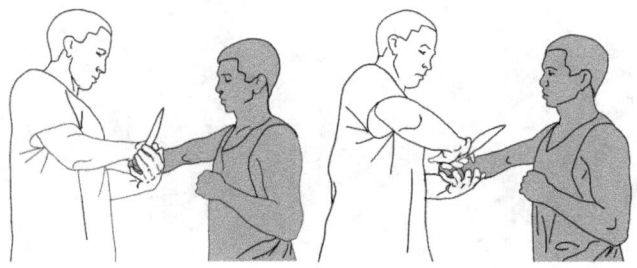

B3

Your opponent attacks with a right straight thrust. Defend using a right chop and a left overhand grab.

Bring your right arm underneath your left arm. The picture is exaggerated for demonstration purposes. You will probably not need to put your hand so close to your armpit.

Use your arm as a guide as you chop the back of your opponent's right hand. The purpose of this is to bend his wrist down.

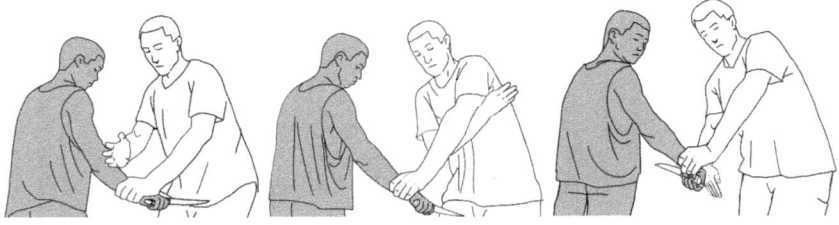

Bend your opponent's arm up and toward him. As you do this, change the grip of your right hand so that your palm is on the back of your opponent's hand.

Apply pressure on your opponent's wrist (toward the outside of his guard) to cause pain, and then disarm him.

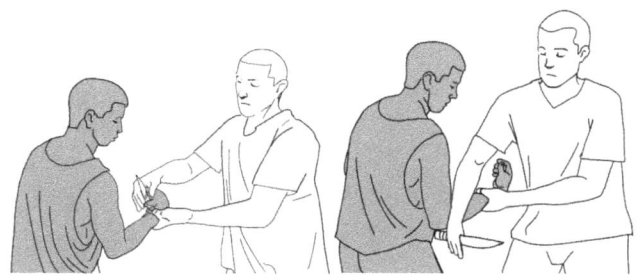

B4

Your opponent attacks with a left straight thrust. Defend using a left chop and right overhand grip.

Bring your left arm underneath your right arm, and then chop down on the back of your opponent's right hand.

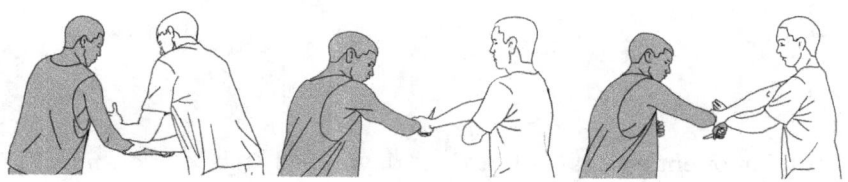

Guide your opponent's right hand to your left. Keep his arm straight. As you do this, grab his wrist with your left hand using an underhand grip. Continue the motion until his elbow faces up.

Shift your left hand from your opponent's wrist to the back of his hand.

Apply pressure to his wrist to cause pain, and then take the knife.

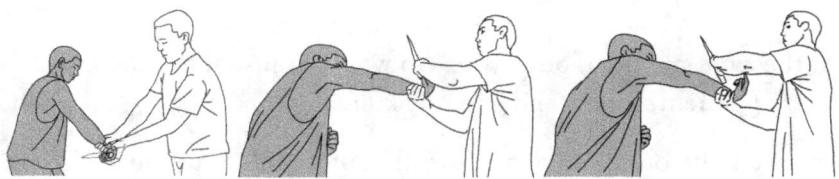

GROUP C

The techniques in group C cause the knife hand to cross from one side of your body to the other. The pattern used is:

1. Block/grab.
2. Disarm.

C1

Your opponent strikes with a right downward stab. As you move to the outside of his guard defend with a left Bong Sau and a right overhand grip. Curve your left arm over your opponent's right arm.

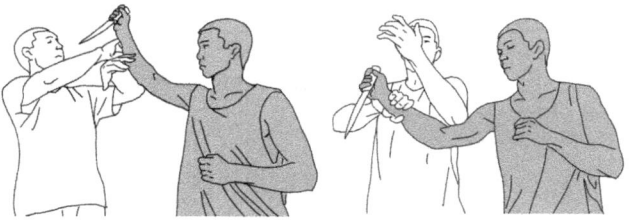

At the right moment, push your elbow down just above the crook of your opponent's elbow and grab the knife.

Pry the knife out of your opponent's hand, pulling to the outside of his guard.

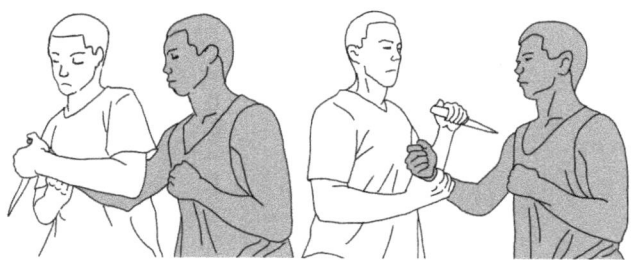

C2

Your opponent attacks with a left downward stab. Defend with a left chop and a right underhand grab.

Bend your opponent's right arm by applying downward pressure to the crook of his elbow with your left hand.

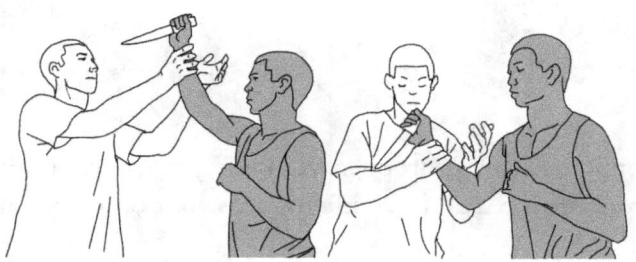

Grab the knife and pry it out of your opponent's hand, pulling toward the outside of his guard.

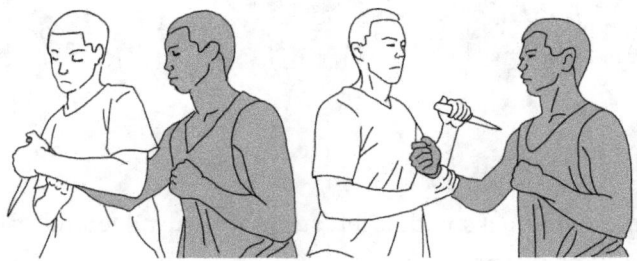

C3

Your opponent attacks with a right straight thrust. Defend with a right chop and a left overhand grab.

Bring your opponent's hand between your two bodies and to your right side.

As you do this, take an overhand grip on your opponent's right wrist with your right hand. Bring your left arm underneath it, perpendicular to his right arm.

The crook of your elbow should be underneath your opponent's elbow. Apply quick pressure by pulling back on his wrist while pushing on his elbow with your left upper arm.

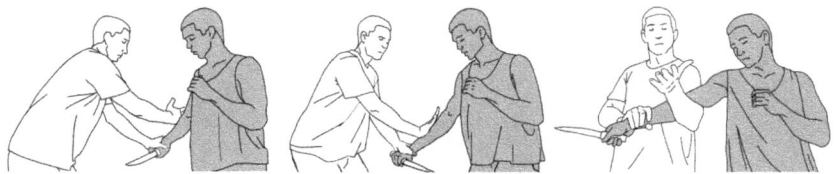

If your opponent hasn't dropped the knife yet, use your left hand to grip it from the top. Pull the knife towards your opponent and out of his grip.

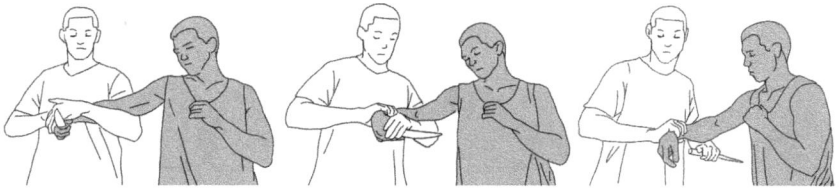

C4

Your opponent attacks with a left straight thrust. Defend using a left chop and right overhand grip.

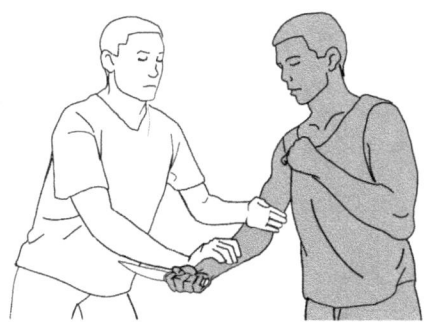

Curl your left arm underneath your opponent's right arm so it is perpendicular to it.

The crook of your elbow should be underneath your opponent's elbow. Apply quick pressure by pulling back on his wrist while pushing on his elbow with your left upper arm.

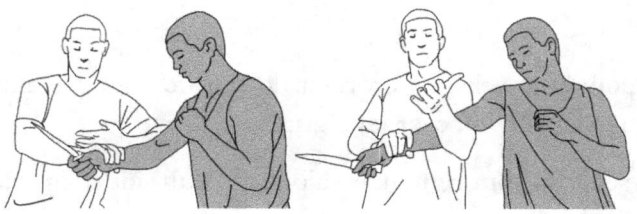

If your opponent hasn't dropped the knife yet, use your left hand to grip it from the top.

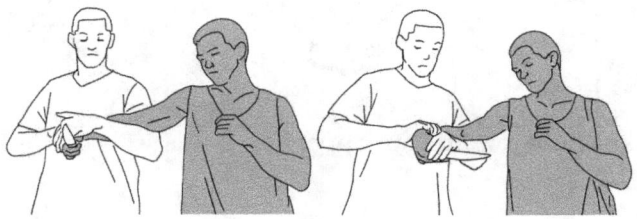

Pull the knife towards your opponent and out of his grip.

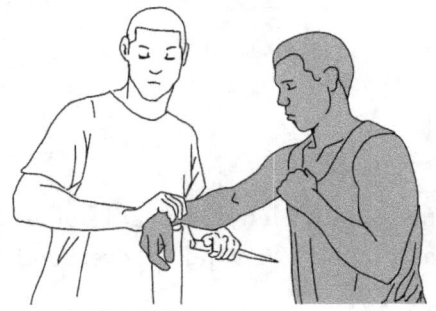

GROUP D

Group D techniques are ones you can do no matter which foot you use to step in first.

D1

Your opponent attacks with a right downward stab. Defend using a right Bong Sau and left overhand grip.

Place the edge of your right hand along the dull side of his blade.

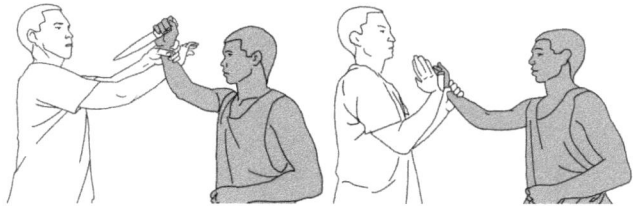

Pull the knife out toward your opponent.

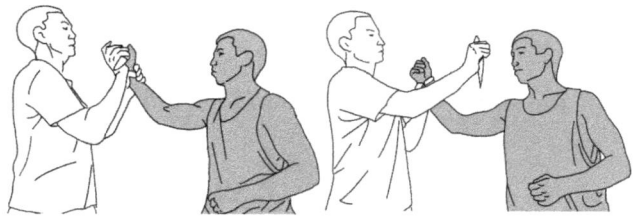

D2

Your opponent attacks with a left downward stab. Defend in the same way as D1, using a right Bong Sau and left overhand grip.

Place the edge of your right hand along the dull side of his blade.

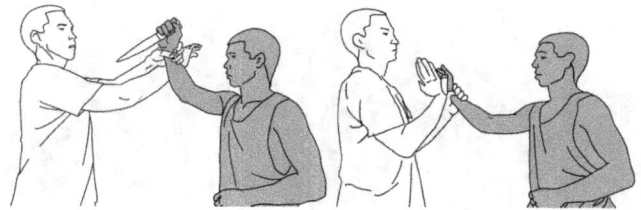

Pull the knife out toward your opponent.

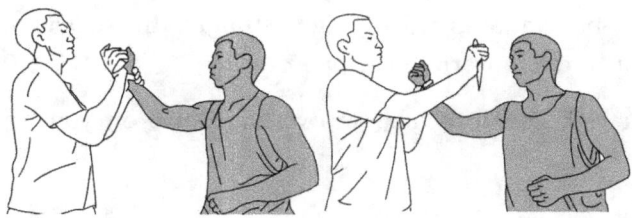

D3 (A)

Your opponent attacks with a right straight thrust. Defend with a left chop and right overhand grip, and then take an overhand grip with your left hand as well.

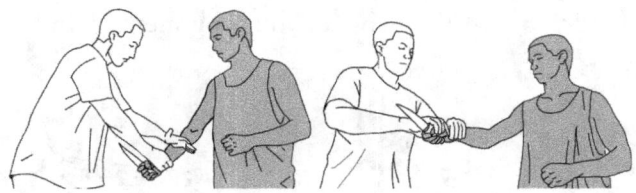

Use your right hand to apply pressure to your opponent's wrist. Release the pressure and then pry the knife out of your opponent's hand, pulling it toward him.

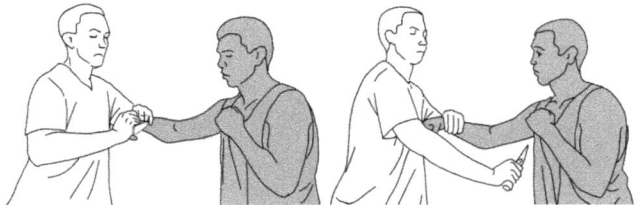

D3 (B)

Your opponent attacks with a right straight thrust. Defend with a right chop and left overhand grip.

Use your right hand to take an overhand grip on your opponent's arm.

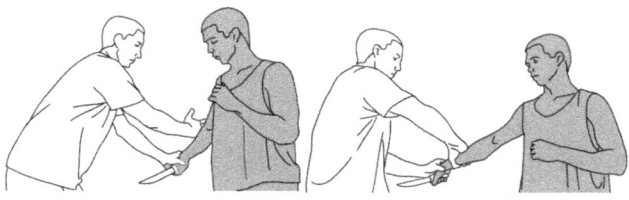

Twist your opponent's arm clockwise, so that his elbow faces up. Use you left hand to pry the knife out of your opponent's hand.

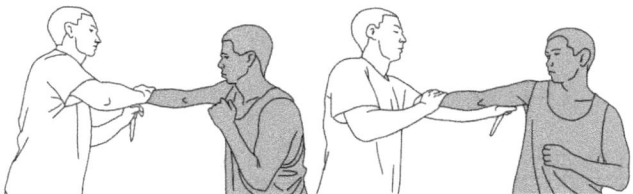

D4 (A)

Your opponent attacks with a left straight thrust. Defend using a right chop and left underhand grip. Adopt an overhand grip on your opponent's wrist with your right hand.

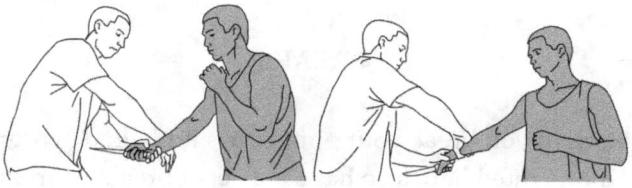

Twist your opponent's arm clockwise, so that his elbow faces up. Use your left hand to pry the knife out of your opponent's hand.

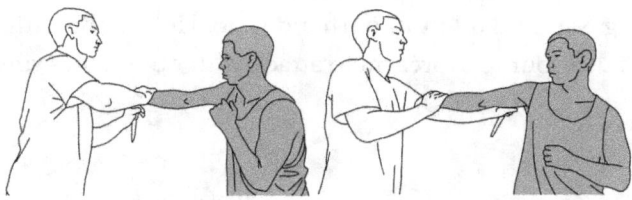

D4 (B)

Your opponent attacks with a left straight thrust. Defend using a left chop and right overhand grip.

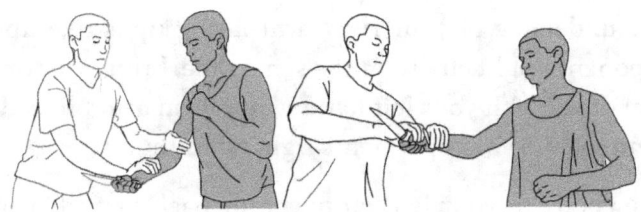

Adopt an overhand grip on your opponent's wrist with your left hand. Use your right hand to apply pressure to your opponent's wrist. Release the pressure and then pry the knife out of your opponent's hand, pulling it toward him.

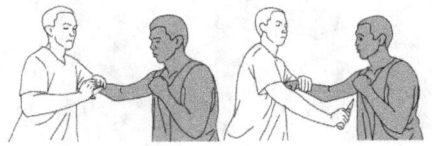

BREAKS

A break is when you break your opponent's limb. Each group of techniques demonstrated here also has a subset of break techniques.

A1 Break

Your opponent attacks with a right overhand stab. Defend with a right Bong Sau and a left underhand grab. Hold tight with your left hand and use your left forearm to attack your opponent's ribs.

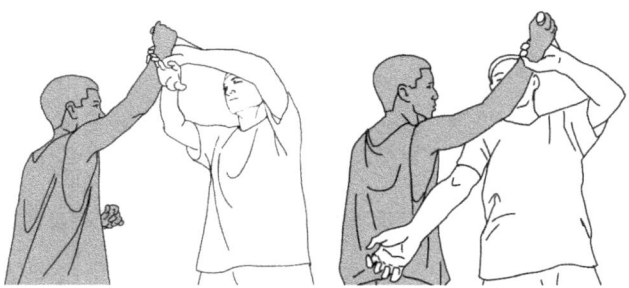

With the underside of your right arm facing up, strike upwards at your opponent's right elbow. At the same time, bring your opponent's right arm down with your left hand to apply an arm break. Use your right hand to grab your opponent's right hand/thumb.

Turn your body to your left, putting your back towards your opponent as you bring his right elbow over your shoulder. Apply pressure downwards to perform a second arm break.

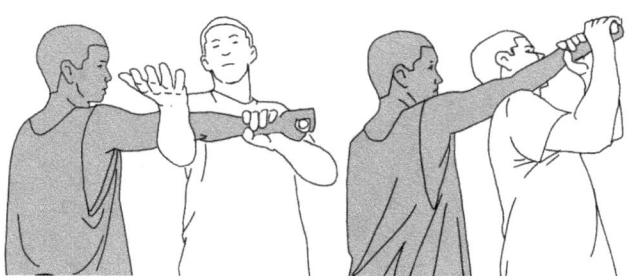

A2 Break

Your opponent attacks with a left downward stab. Use a left chop and a right overhand grip to defend.

Simultaneously use your right hand to twist your opponent's right hand and let your left forearm fall on your opponent's arm in a waterfall action (see the Principles of Self-Defense chapter). This will twist his elbow to face up and straighten his arm out at the same time.

Apply downward pressure to your opponent's elbow.

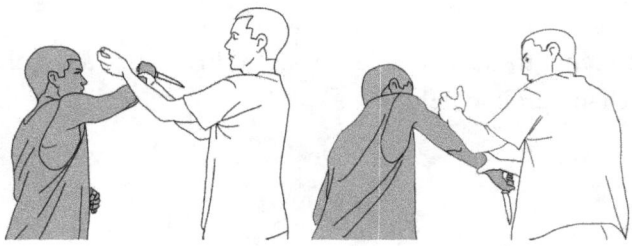

A3 Break

Your opponent attacks with a right straight stab. Defend using a right chop and a left overhand grab.

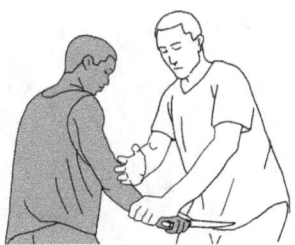

Step back with your right foot as you bring your opponent's right hand across your body. As you do this, adopt an overhand grip with your right hand.

Step in with your left leg and use your left forearm to strike/apply pressure on your opponent's right elbow.

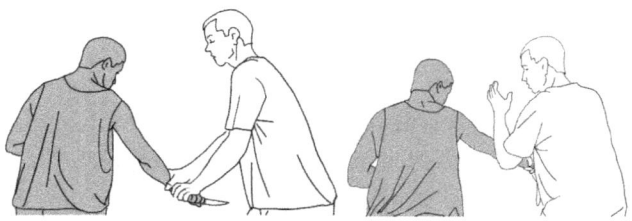

A4 Break

Your opponent attacks with a left straight thrust. Use a left chop and a right overhand grab to defend.

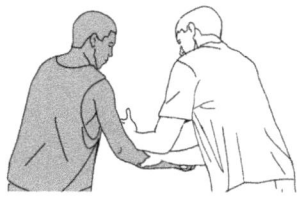

Pull your opponent's arm back and across your body to straighten it out. At the same time, bring your left arm back to create some space between it (your left arm) and your opponent's right arm.

Use your left forearm to strike/apply pressure on your opponent's right elbow.

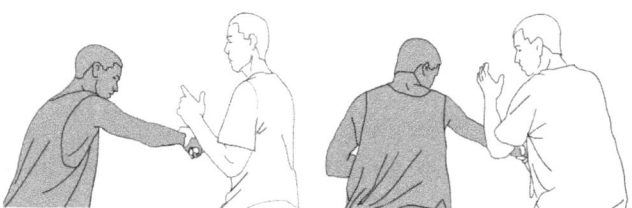

B1 Break

All B breaks use an overhand grip and the same arm-break technique.

Your opponent attacks with a right downward stab. Defend with a left Bong Sau and a right overhand grab.

Guide your opponent's right arm down as you shift your body to the outside of his guard.

As your opponent's right arm comes down, bring your right hand up on the inside of his guard. The intention is to grab your opponent's hand so he cannot let go of the knife.

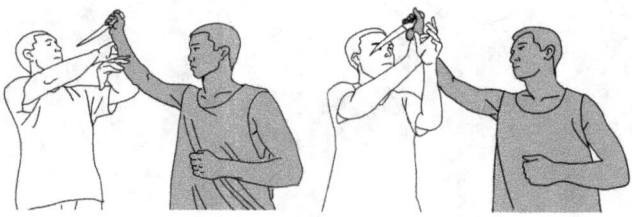

Continue to guide your opponent's arm down until it's horizontal and tight across your body. Your opponent's arm should sit snugly in the crook of your elbow.

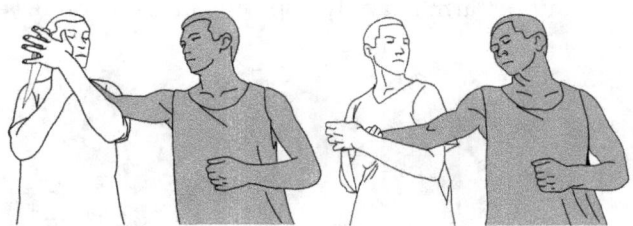

Apply the break by pulling your opponent's hand towards you while using your left upper arm to apply opposing pressure on his elbow.

B2 Break

Your opponent attacks with a left downward stab. Defend with a left chop and a right underhand grab. You could also use a left Bong Sao.

Guide your opponent's right arm down as you shift your body to the outside of his guard.

As your opponent's right arm comes down, curl your left hand underneath it. The intention is to grab your opponent's hand so he cannot let go of the knife.

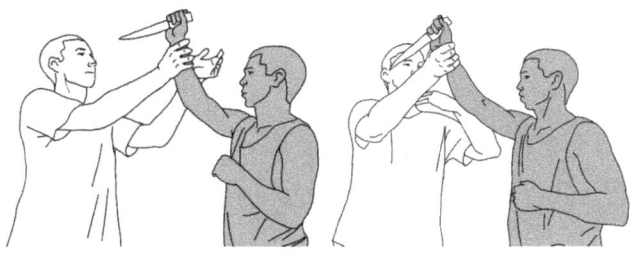

Continue to guide your opponent's arm down until it's horizontal and tight across your body. Your opponent's arm should sit snugly in the crook of your elbow.

Apply the break by pulling your opponent's hand towards you while using your left upper arm to apply opposing pressure on his elbow.

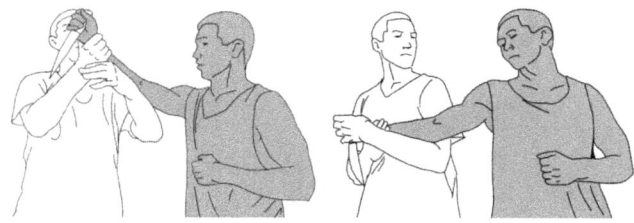

B3 Break

Your opponent attacks with a right straight thrust. Defend with a right chop and a left overhand grab.

Guide your opponent's right hand between your bodies.

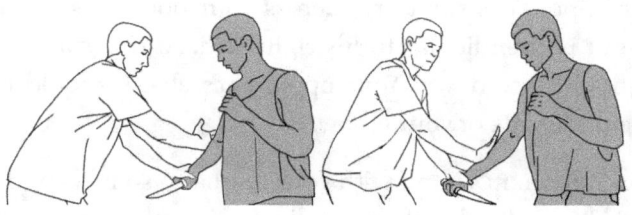

As you do this, use adopt an overhand grip on his right hand with *your* right hand, so he cannot let go of the knife.

Continue to guide your his arm between the two of you until it is horizontal and tight across your body. It should sit snugly in the crook of your elbow.

Apply the break by pulling your opponent's hand towards you whilst using your left upper arm to apply opposing pressure on his elbow.

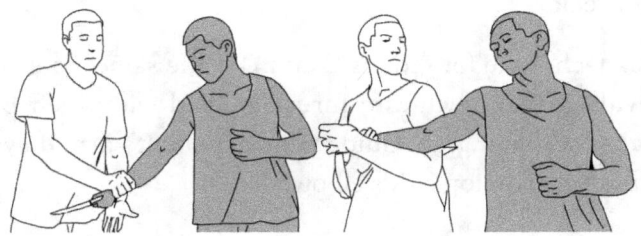

B4 Break

Your opponent attacks with a left straight thrust. Defend with a left Bong Sau and a right overhand grab. You could also use a left chop.

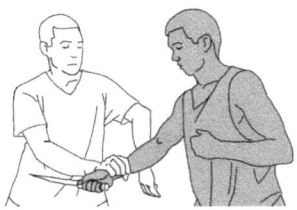

Pull your opponent's right arm across your body as straighten your left arm out perpendicular to his right arm. At this stage, both your elbows should face down. Your opponent's elbow should be on the top of the underside of your elbow.

Grab your opponent's hand with your left hand so he cannot let go of the knife. Apply the break by pulling his hand towards you while using your left upper arm to apply opposing pressure to his elbow.

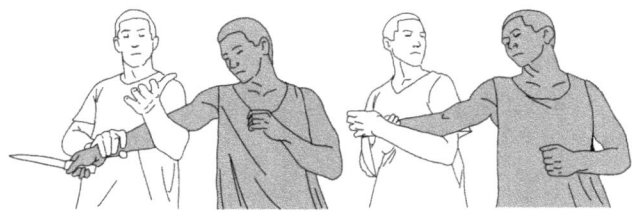

C and D Breaks

The break technique for groups C and D is the same. Your opponent attacks with a right downward thrust. Defend with a left Bong Sau and a right overhand grab. Guide your opponent's arm down as you curl your left arm on top of his elbow.

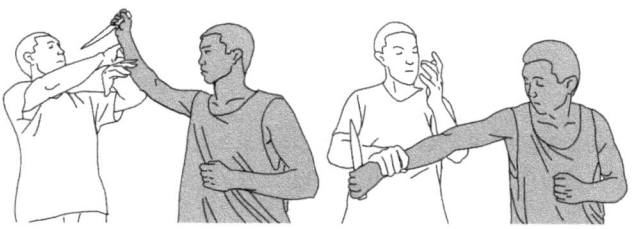

Using a waterfall technique with your left forearm, force your opponent down.

Use your left hand to hold your opponent's shoulder. Place your knee on top of your opponent's elbow and apply downward pressure while pulling up at his wrist and shoulder.

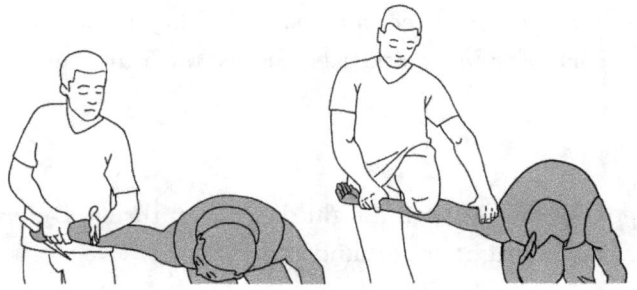

Related Chapters:

- Principles of Self-Defense

UNIVERSALS

Universals are disarming techniques that you can use at any time, no matter what foot you step in with, which block and/or grab you use, or what the angle of attack is.

There are two universal techniques. The following demonstrations show how each of them can be used against the four angles of attack.

Universals 1A

Your opponent attacks with a right downward thrust. Defend with a left Bong Sau and right underhand grab.

Guide your opponent's arm down as you curl your left hand towards you and then overtop of his upper arm. At this point, you may choose to strike him in the face.

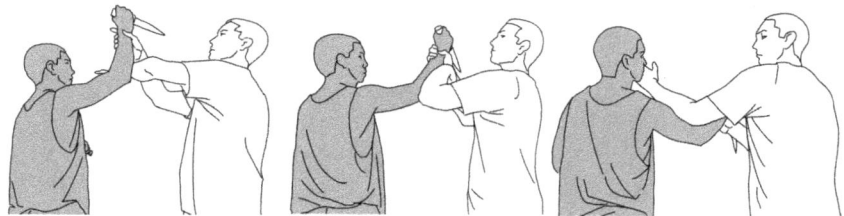

Continue to hook down inside your opponent's guard with your left arm until you grab your own right forearm.

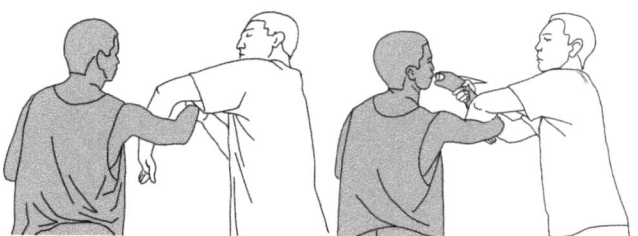

Drive your right elbow into your opponent's face, and then grip the top of the knife with your left hand.

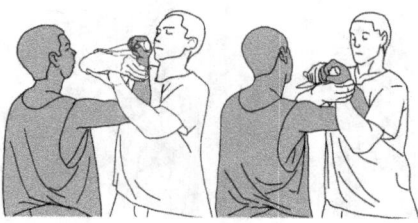

Release your right hand and move it away so you can pry the knife out of your opponent's hand, pulling it toward the outside of his guard.

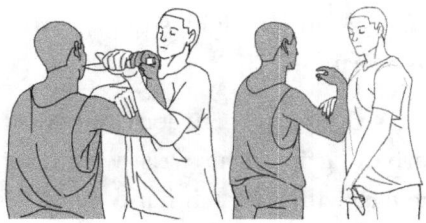

Universals 1B

Your opponent attacks with a left downward thrust. Defend with a left chop and right underhand grip.

Use your left hand to strike your opponent.

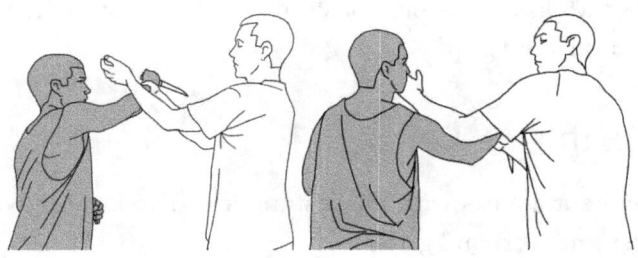

Continue to hook down inside your opponent's guard with your left arm until you grab your own right forearm.

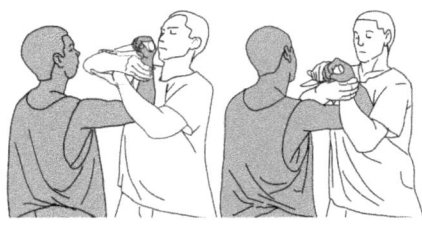

Continue the disarm as previously described.

Universals 1C

Your opponent attacks with a right straight thrust. Defend with a right chop and left overhand grip.

Pass your opponent's right arm between your two bodies. As you do this, adopt an overhand grip on his wrist with your right hand while striking him in the face with your left hand.

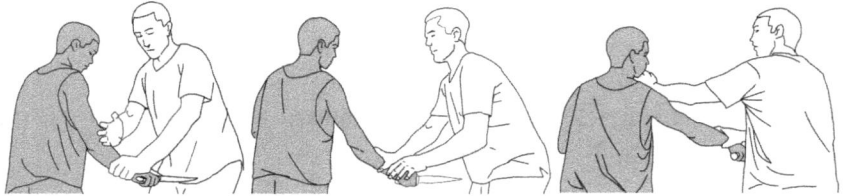

Continue the disarm as previously described. Your right hand can stay in an overhand grip.

Universals 1D

Your opponent attacks with a left straight thrust. Defend with a left chop and right overhand grip.

Use your right hand to raise your opponent's arm a little so you can curl your left arm under.

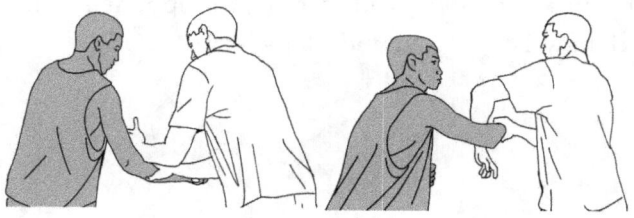

Perform the disarm as previously described.

Universals 2A

Your opponent attacks with a right downward stab. Defend using a left Bong Sau and a right underhand grip. As you guide your opponent's arm down, curl your left arm so it ends up on top of his right elbow.

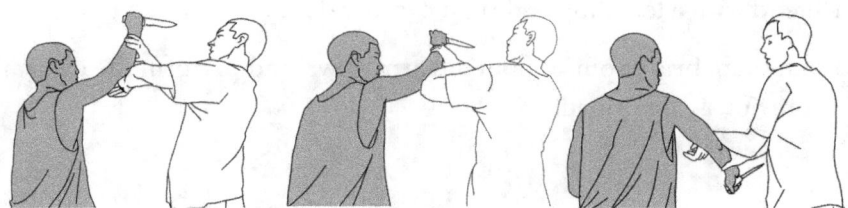

Pass your left hand between your opponent's arm and torso to grab the back of his shoulder. At the same time, move your opponent's arm back with your right hand, so that you stay clear of the knife.

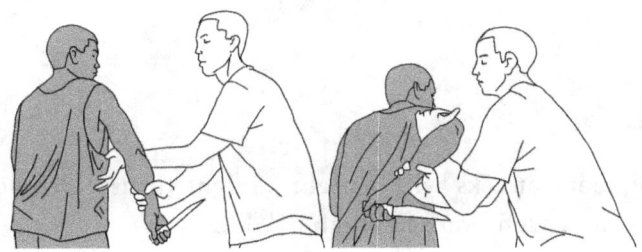

Use your left hand to apply downward pressure on your opponent's shoulder and lock it in place.

Let go of your right hand. Bring it over your opponent's shoulder and grab his right wrist using an underhand grip.

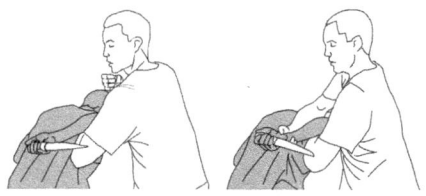

Pull your opponent's wrist towards his right shoulder to apply the lock/break and then take the knife.

Universals 2B

Your opponent attacks with a left downward stab.

Defend with a left chop and right overhand grip.

From there bring your opponent's arm down and perform the disarm as previously described.

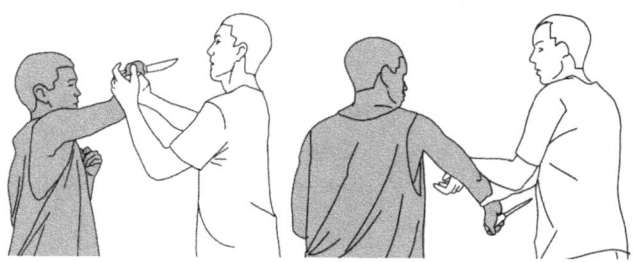

Universals 2C

Your opponent attacks with a right straight thrust. Defend with a right chop and a left overhand grab.

Step to your left so that you're on the outside of your opponent's guard. As you do this, adopt an overhand grip on your opponent's wrist with your right hand.

Once you have a good grip with your left hand, use your right arm to pass between your opponent's arm and body.

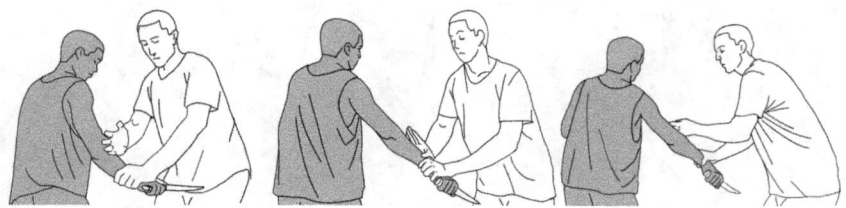

Continue to apply the disarm as previously described.

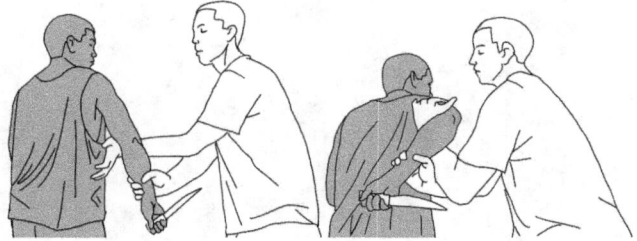

Universals 2D

Your opponent attacks with a left straight thrust. Defend using a left chop and right overhand grab.

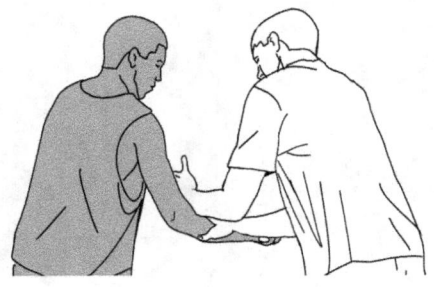

Pass your left arm between your opponent's arm and body, and then continue to apply the disarm as previously described.

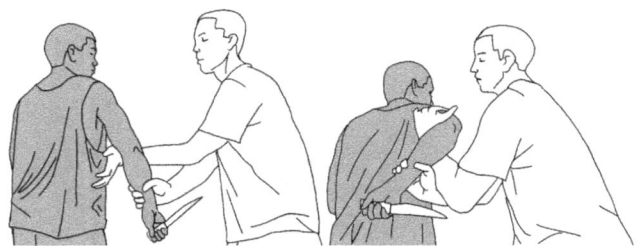

SELF-KILLS

Self-kill techniques are those in which you use the attacker's knife against him while the knife is still in his hand.

This way, you can tell the authorities that you never even touched the knife. He pulled it on you, there was a messy struggle, and he ended up getting hurt.

The label "self-kill" does not mean you have to kill your opponent. A shallow stab in a superficial area will be enough to finish most confrontations.

Self-Kill 1

Your opponent attacks with a right downward stab. Defend using a right Bong Sau and left underhand grab.

Use your right hand to grab your opponent's right wrist with an underhand grip. Facilitate this by bending your opponent's right upper arm to the outside of his guard with your left hand.

Once you have a good grip with your right hand, place your left hand over your opponent's hand so he will not be able to let go of the knife.

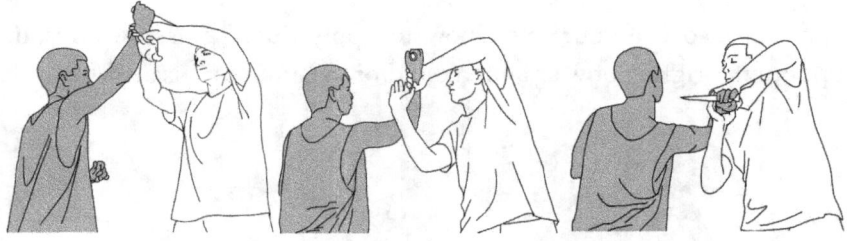

Drive the knife into your opponent's neck. If needed, you can grab the other side of your opponent's neck and pull it into the knife.

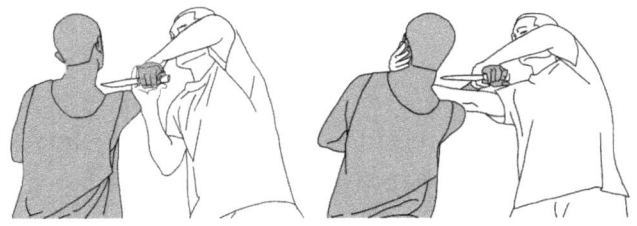

Self-Kill 2

Your opponent attacks with a left downward stab. Defend using a left chop and right underhand grab.

Use your left hand to grab over your opponent's right hand with an overhand grip so that he cannot let go of the knife.

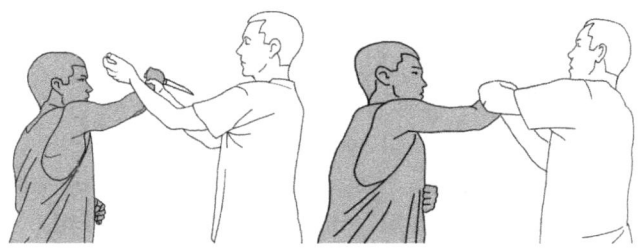

Once you have a good grip, turn the knife towards your opponent and stab him with it.

You can also use your left elbow to apply quick pressure on your opponent's right elbow as a break and/or to soften up his arm.

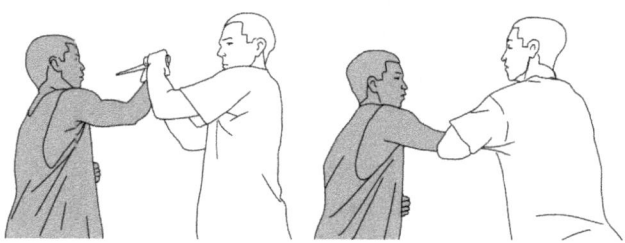

Self-Kill 3

Your opponent attacks with a right straight thrust. Defend using a right chop and left overhand grab.

Use your right hand to grab hold of your opponent's wrist and then move your left hand over his hand. Bend your opponent's wrist down.

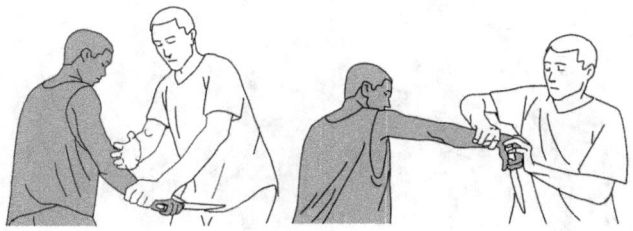

Pull up on your opponent's wrist while pushing his hand down and toward his side.

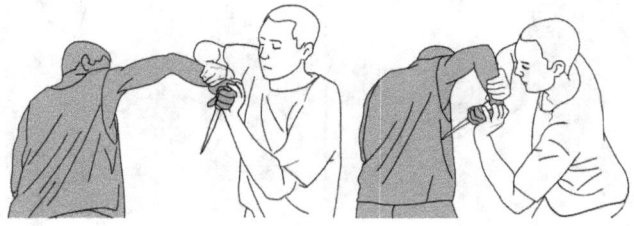

Self-Kill 4

Your opponent attacks with a left straight thrust. Defend using a left chop and right underhand grip.

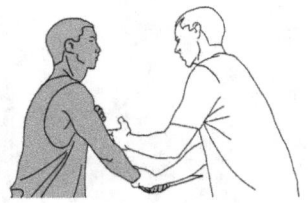

Grab your opponent's hand with your left hand using an overhand grip. Once you have a good grip, move your right hand over the same hand. Your two hands ensure your opponent cannot let go of the knife.

Pull your opponent's arm to the outside of your right shoulder and then fold his wrist back towards him. This will cause his arm to bend so you can slash or stab him.

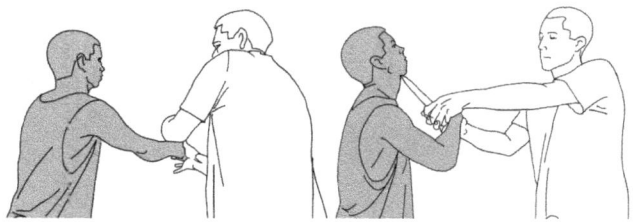

Alternatively, you could also perform a wrist lock.

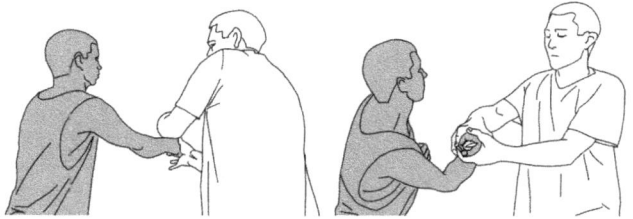

Related Chapters:

- Attack

KNIFE FLOW DRILL

It is best if you are at least familiar with all the different disarms described so far before progressing to this knife flow drill.

One person (P1) has a knife and attacks from any angle he chooses. The other person (P2) practices his block/grab defense. P1 then practices countering the block/grab defense. Once free, P1 can then attack again, either from the same angle or a different one.

The countering of the block/grab is the new concept in this drill. P2 should allow P1 to perform the action to begin with. When ready, P2 can start to make things harder by disarming P1 if he is too slow to counter.

There is no set pattern to this drill. The following is just an example of what could happen. When first learning the knife flow drill, you may wish to copy this example, but as you progress, you will learn to instinctively choose the best action in your situation.

P1 attacks with a right downward stab. P2 defends using a left Bong Sau and right underhand grip.

P2 curls his left forearm underneath and then on top of P1's arm, and then grabs his knife-wielding hand.

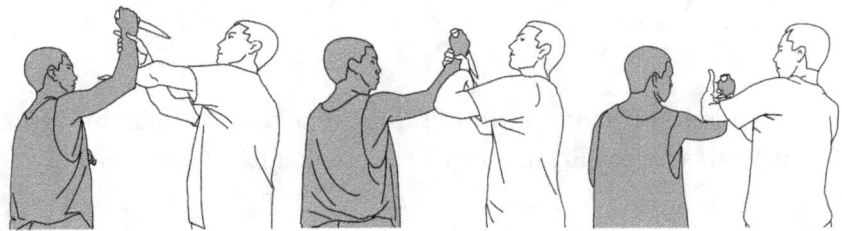

P1 uses his left hand to push on P2's elbow and free his hand.

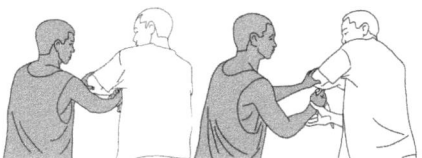

P1 attacks with a left downward stab. P2 defends with a left chop and right underhand grab. P2 uses his left hand to grab P1's thumb and then twists it to the outside of P1's guard.

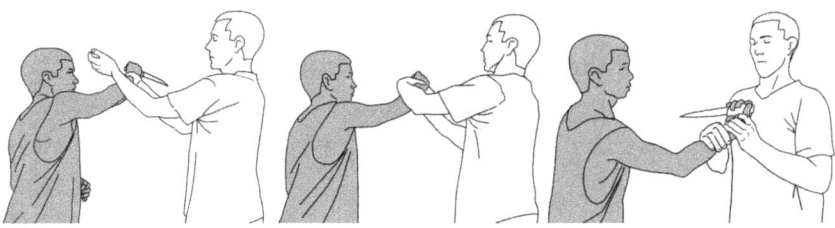

P1 pushes up on P2's right wrist to free his hand. P1 attacks with a right straight thrust. P2 defends with a right chop and left underhand grab.

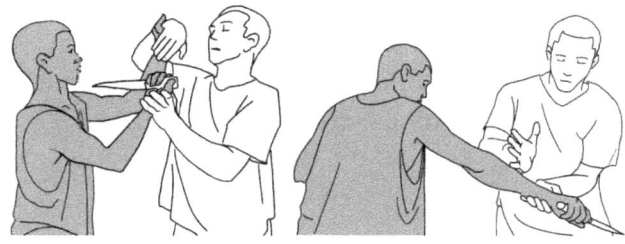

P2 uses his right hand to grab P1's right hand and bends his wrist down. P2 then twists P1's arm clockwise, so that his elbow is facing up.

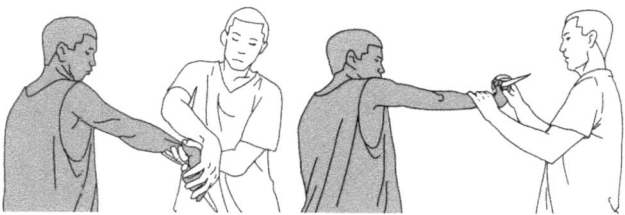

P1 uses his left hand to push up on P2's wrist to free his hand. P1 attacks with a left straight thrust. P2 defends with a left chop and right underhand grab.

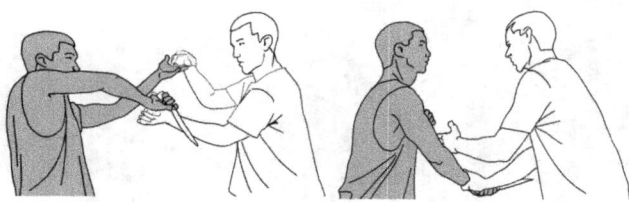

P2 grabs P1's hand with his left hand and applies a wrist lock by twisting P1's arm to the outside of his guard.

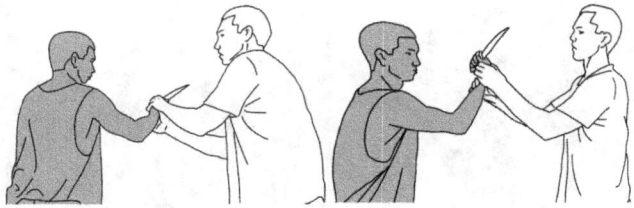

Before the lock is applied, P1 pushes up on P2's right hand to release the grip.

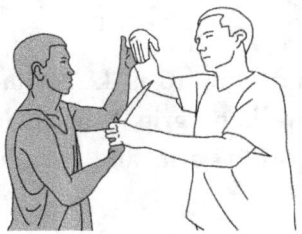

The rest of this demonstration shows some alternative flows focusing on the first strike—that is, a downward right stab. This same idea can be applied to any strike/defense/counter. It's presented here just to give you an idea of how you can adapt this drill in training.

P1 attacks with a right downward strike again. P2 defends with a left Bong Sau and right overhand grip. P2 uses his right hand to grab P1's right thumb and begins to bring it down.

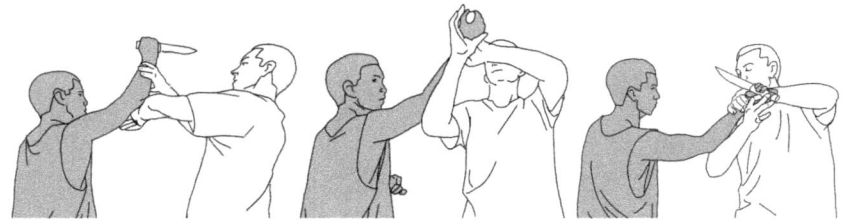

P1 hits down on his own right arm at the crook of his elbow to escape the hold.

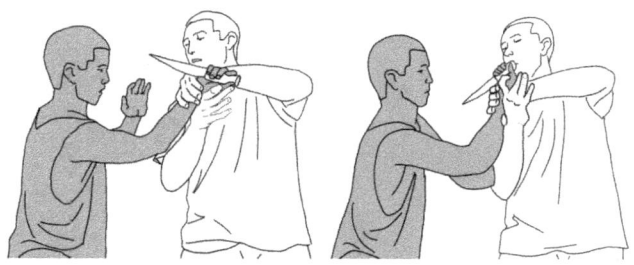

Note: If P2 uses a proper grip and continues into Self Kill 1, P1 will probably not be able to do this reversal.

P1 attacks with a right downward strike again. P2 defends with a left Bong Sau and right overhand grip. P2 curls his left forearm underneath and then on top of P1's arm, and then grabs his knife-wielding hand.

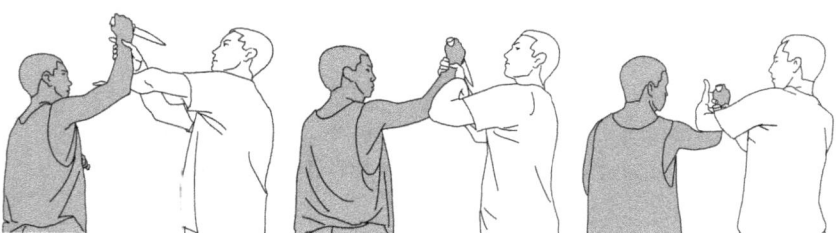

P1 uses his left hand to push on P2's elbow to free his hand.

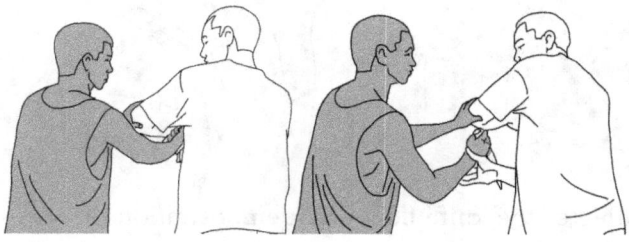

P2 then uses his left hand to grab P2's left arm and applies an arm break.

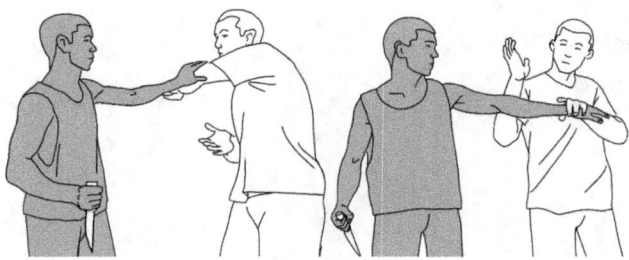

P1 attacks with a right downward strike again and P2 catches P1's wrist with his right hand.

P2 brings his right hand over P1's right arm to apply a lock.

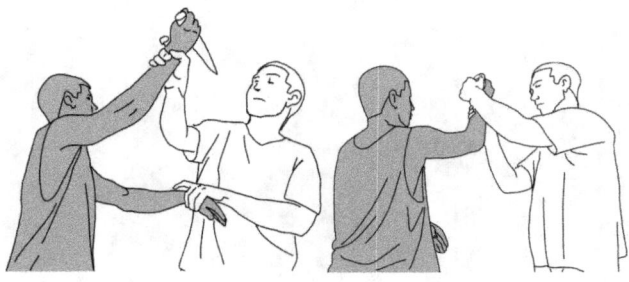

P1 pushes up at P2's left wrist to release his arm.

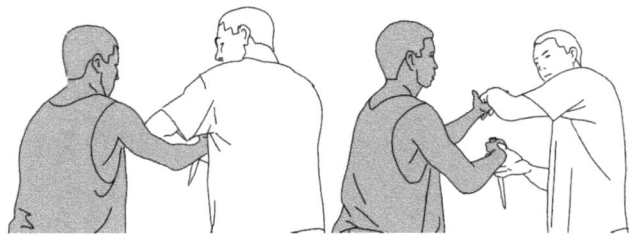

This completes the knife flow drill demonstration. As you may realize, it has infinite variations.

Related Chapters:

- Attack
- Defense

BONUS CHAPTERS

The following bonus chapters are direct excerpts from *The Self-Defense Handbook* by Sam Fury.

www.SFNonfictionBooks.com/Self-Defense-Handbook

IMPROVISED WEAPONS

When running isn't an option, and you have the opportunity to get one, use a weapon.

If you can hit with, thrust, throw, spray, or hide behind something, it's a potential improvised weapon. That covers almost any object, though some are better than others.

A good improvised weapon is one that you can carry around without suspicion—that is, one a police officer would not take off you in the street. Examples of such weapons are:

- An umbrella
- A pen
- Hairspray and a lighter (for a makeshift flamethrower)

There are four types of improvised weapons that are the best to use for self-defense:

- Knives
- Clubs
- Shields
- Projectiles

When training with improvised weapons, choose things you routinely carry around, like an umbrella, a pen, or trade tools.

The generic grip for any weapon is to hold it firmly in your fist, but not so tightly that doing so causes fatigue. Put your legs in an aggressive ready stance.

Knives

Knives are one-handed thrusting objects. Besides an actual knife, you could use a bottle, scissors, a rolled-up magazine, etc.

Hold the knife in your strong hand and use a weak lead.

Position your knife hand down and back at your waist. Use your lead hand to guard.

Thrust straight out at your opponent's abdomen and bring your arm straight back

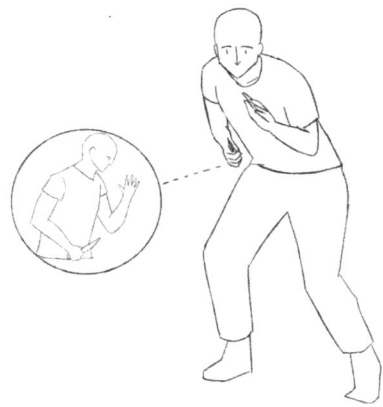

Clubs

A club can be any solid object that is too big to be a knife, but not so big that it's cumbersome. A metal pipe, a baseball bat, a walking stick, etc., are all good clubs.

Hold your club in both hands, up behind your shoulder. Alternatively, hold it in one hand and use the other as a guard.

Strike straight down into your opponent's head, and/or thrust the club into his face or gut.

You can also strike his knee, which is a less damaging target, but will still put him out of commission.

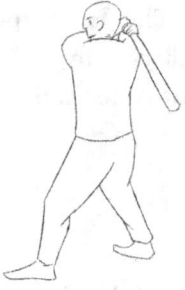

Shields

Anything you can hide behind or use as an obstacle—a chair, a door, a wall, a backpack, etc.— makes a good shield.

If you can pick it up, use it to block and thrust. If it's an immovable object, ram your opponent's head into it.

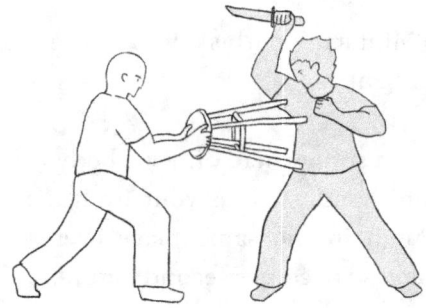

Projectiles

A projectile is anything you can throw or spray that isn't better used some other way, such as an ashtray, deodorant, hot liquid, or dirt.

Tactical Pen

A tactical pen is a good example of a knife weapon that you can carry around without suspicion. The best type of tactical pen for self-defense is one that you'll carry. Any simple stainless-steel pen will work, but ideally, you'll choose one that:

- Is refillable
- Writes well (you like it)
- Has a clip
- Has a flat top (that won't stab you)
- Is easy to replace/inexpensive
- Can pass as a normal pen (to get through security)

Most of the tactical pens on the market do not fill these requirements, especially the last one. Those that do include:

- Zebra 701
- Zebra 402
- Parker Jotter
- Fisher Space Military Pen (this one is a little more expensive, but still under $20)

Clip your tactical pen somewhere on your body that is easy to access with your dominant hand, such as your front pants pocket on your dominant side. Put it in the same place every time and practice deploying it, so doing so becomes second nature.

When you grab the pen, hold it in an icepick grip, with your thumb on top.

Every time you initially grab the pen, including to write something or to put it away, use this grip.

Grab the pen and thrust it straight into your opponent in one swift movement. A cardboard box makes a good target when training.

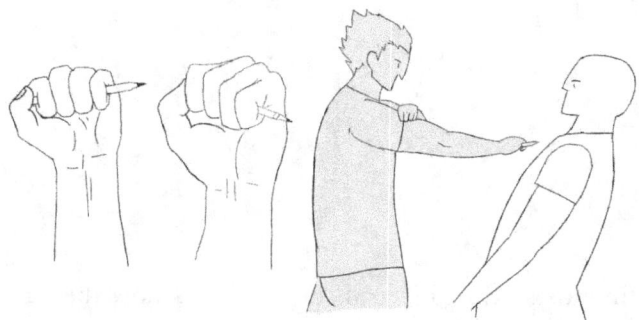

You can strike from almost any angle. Thrust the pen into any target area to help you escape.

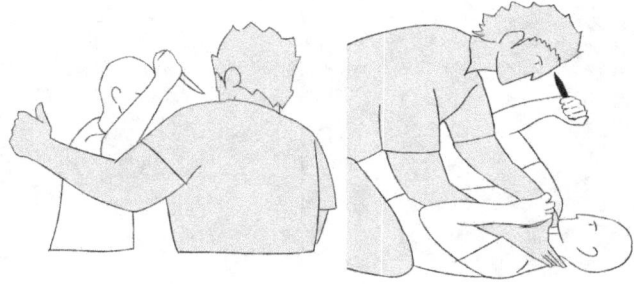

Sap

Anything heavy in a sock makes a good improvised sap. You can use coins, a billiard ball, a soda can, or a rock.

Another way to make one is to tie a metal nut (or something similar) to a piece of cord, such as a shoelace.

A piece of material about the size of a tea towel (or t-shirt) with a small weighted object (like a handful of coins) in it also works.

- Put the object in the center of the material.
- Fold the material diagonally in half over the object.
- Roll up the material from the point to the base.

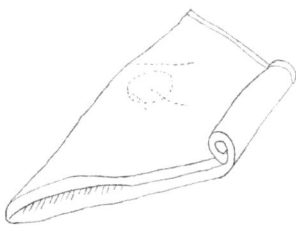

Hold both ends so the object in the middle is now the striking end. Use it like a club—that is, make vertical strikes to your opponent's head. You can also uppercut.

WEAPON VS WEAPON

If you're going to fight someone with a weapon, getting your own weapon will give you the best chance of success.

In addition to the following information, review the improvised weapons chapter.

Your opponent's hand makes a good secondary target if it's closer than his head.

When using a knife, use timing, footwork, and feints. Wait for your opponent to strike and then close in before he can recover. You can use a feint to time his strike.

If you have a club, use the overhead strike straight down along the central line. If your opponent uses an angled attack, your straight overhead will win. When you both use the overhead strike, the strike that hits its target first will succeed.

If your opponent's strike is going to beat yours, parry it. As his strike comes in, tap the top of your weapon on his to deflect it. Immediately return your club to the center line to finish your strike.

When you hold a longer weapon, keep the advantage of distance. Use footwork, overhead strikes, and thrusts.

Related Chapters:

- Attack
- Improvised Weapons

PART III

STICK FIGHTING

EXPLANATION OF TERMS

The following terms are specific to stick fighting.

Changing Grip

Changing grip (a.k.a. switching grip) means shifting from an overhand grip on your opponent's stick to an underhand one. Doing this will make it easier to perform certain actions. Whichever way your palm faces is the direction that will be easiest for you to push, hence making it easier to snatch.

Note: Snatching is when you disarm your opponent. It is explained in detail later on in this book.

This means, assuming your opponent is in a structurally correct position, you can anticipate what he will do by noting the direction his palm faces.

The best way to change grip is to first push the stick into your opponent's face.

This will cause him pain and will also bring you to his center, which will make it harder for him to move back.

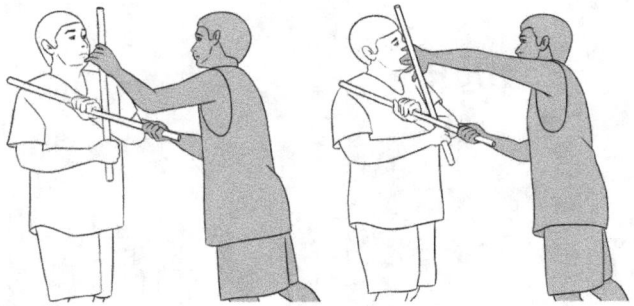

When grabbing low, it is preferable to use an underhand grip. You can snatch more easily, and the grip exposes your muscle rather than your bone, so if your opponent hits your arm it will not hurt as much.

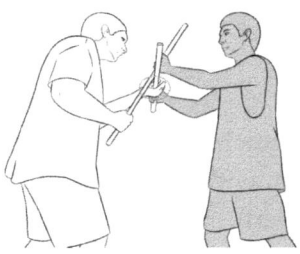

Jumping Hands

Jumping hands is moving your hand from a high position on your opponent's stick to a low position, or vice versa. It is necessary to do this in order to create opportunities for yourself or to prevent your opponent from snatching your stick.

If you just try to jump from high to low, or vice versa, your opponent can pull his stick back, so that you miss. To prevent this, push your opponent's, stick towards him a little before jumping. The natural reaction of your opponent will be to push back because he will not want to get hit in the face. Make the jump when your opponent does this push back.

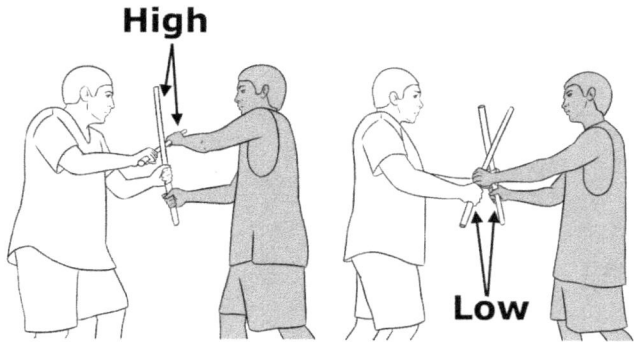

BASIC STANCE

When stationary, stand with your feet a bit wider than shoulder width apart. Hold the stick in your strongest hand and have your strong side as your lead. The bottom of your weapon should extend between one and two inches below your little finger. Unless you're performing an action (attack or defense), hold your stick back over your shoulder. Your hand should be near your ear on the same side, and the tip of your weapon should point to your rear. Doing this will:

- keep your hand out of range of your opponent's strike (if he hits your hand you might drop your weapon; and
- give your strikes the greatest power and speed for attacking your primary target—namely your opponent's head.

Your rear hand is a backup for defense or secondary attack, and should be kept close to your centerline most of the time.

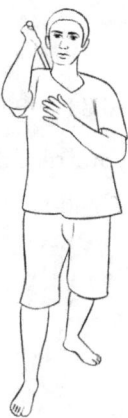

Related Chapters:

- Attack

STEPPING

Advancing with the stick is the same as in hand to hand combat.

Spring semi-forward stepping is used to close distance. In this technique, your back heel is up. This turns your calf muscle into a double spring—one behind your knee and one at your heel. Releasing these springs propels your whole body forward.

Take a small step forward with your lead foot and place your rear foot in the original position of your lead.

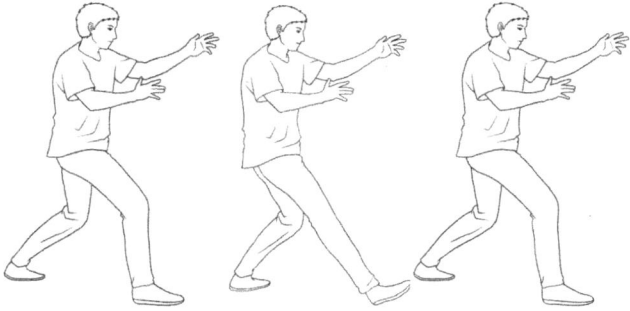

Your stance should never be exaggerated (too long or short).

Keep most of your weight on your rear leg. The heel of your front foot should land first, followed by the toes of both feet. This will keep you well-grounded and ready for the next move.

THE KING OF STRIKES

In Kali Arnis, each strike angle is given a number. These number assignments are common to most lineages, including other weapon systems such as Escrima.

When it comes to stick-fighting, the best strike by far is the number seven. In Vortex Control Stick-Fighting, it has been dubbed the "king of strikes" and is the first strike you learn. It is also the one you will use most often.

Strikes one to six come in on angles to hit the meaty parts of your opponent. The number seven strike comes straight down between your eyes. With it, you own the centerline, and whoever owns the centerline has the advantage.

When used offensively, the strike targets your opponent's face or the top of his head. In a defensive capacity, it protects you from any angulated strike. To do the number seven strike, start in the basic stance. Bring your stick straight down the center into your target. As the stick comes down, bring your other hand up. This helps keep you balanced and is also a backup defense.

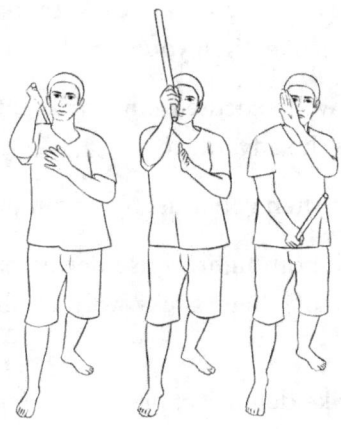

Practice this fundamental strike in a stationary position, with forward stepping, and as double hits.

Simple but very effective combinations can be made all along the number seven axis. Here is one example:

- Double hit, straight thrust, and step though with an uppercut using the bottom of the stick.

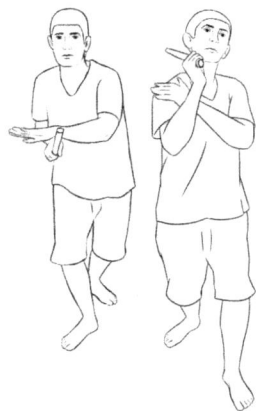

The Seven Defense

If your opponent uses an angled attack (either intentionally or in a poorly executed king strike) then your number seven (king) will win.

When you both use well-executed king strikes, then whoever is first to the target will have the advantage.

If you are not the first, then you must turn your attack into a defense.

Note: Theoretically, if both fighters use perfect number sevens at the same time, the tips of their sticks will clash. In reality, this is extremely unlikely.

To make the king strike defensive, place your rear hand behind your stick as you do the strike.

If needed, you can turn slightly toward the angle your opponent's strike is coming on.

Do not turn more than 10°. It is the creation of triangles that makes the defense structure strong.

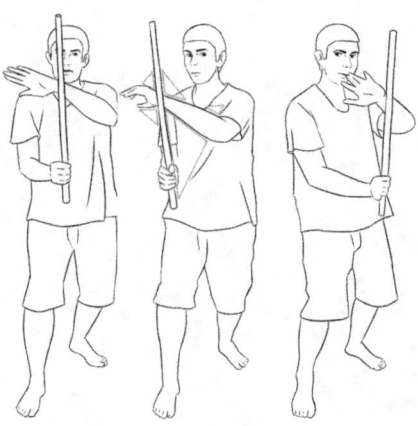

Another way to use the number seven in defense is if you are under pressure—if your opponent is holding your stick down, for example. Just return to a number seven position.

You may need to step back to create space and/or move your weapon in a circular motion to facilitate this.

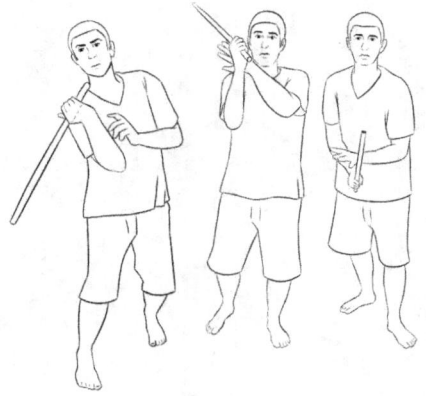

The act of "returning to seven" is a simple and effective strategy to regain dominance, and is referred to more throughout this book.

Related Chapters:

- Attack
- Basic Stance

QUEEN STRIKE

A very important strike in Vortex Control Stick-Fighting is the queen strike.

The queen strike is derived from the abanico movement, as opposed the sword-type movement other strikes, such as the king strike.

Abanico is done by flicking your wrist so your stick follows a fan shape. This movement allows the stick to go around common defenses and strike at unexpected angles.

The queen strike is quicker but less powerful than the king. Its big advantage is that it can be used at close range. While the king is good when you have space, the queen is effective once your opponent moves in close and/or grabs your stick or wrist while your arm is down.

When your opponent grabs you, slap down on his hand and do the queen strike. The slap will pull your opponent into your strike as well as help to flick your strike into his face (left picture).

It is also very easy to defend against a strike from this position, which has the same structure as when you're using the king strike as a defense (right picture).

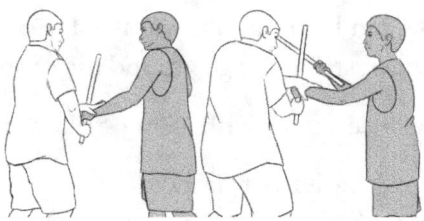

Although you want all strikes to be fast and well-aimed, this is more important with the queen strike. For example, aim for the eye when executing a head shot. You can practice in the air or with a small target by continuously making fast strikes to a single point.

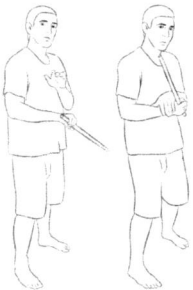

The queen strike can be magnified by dropping into it (grounding). As you do the queen, quickly sink your weight and move back. This will straighten your opponent's arm, throw him off balance, give him a "whiplash" effect, and nullify his other arm.

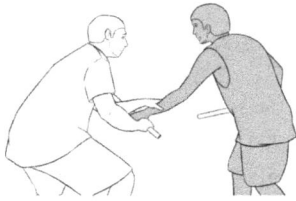

Queen Defense and Counters

Defending against a queen strike is more difficult than with other strikes. The biggest problem is that you need to see the strike coming.

The seven defense can be used, but you need to angulate more than usual, since the queen strike can go around the centerline.

To counter this defense, attack with a king strike as follows.

You (the person on the left) strike with a queen strike while your opponent defends with a modified seven defense.

Use your left hand to cover his arms as you retract your stick and counter with a king strike (returning to seven).

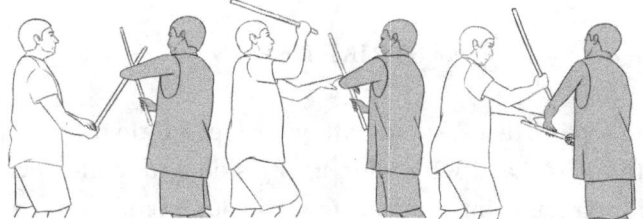

If your stick is on his, you can defend against the queen strike by moving your stick away from your opponent's hand. This will nullify the pivot point his stick moves around. That is, your stick becomes a "wall" as opposed to being part of the pivot point.

To counter this defense, use your hand to hit your opponent's stick in the same direction he is moving it as he creates a gap. Hit it completely off your stick.

Once his stick is out of the way, you'll have many options, such as queen strikes or returning to seven.

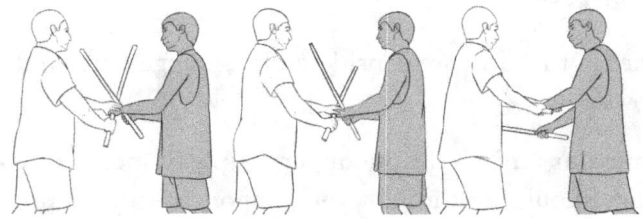

Note: Pushing your opponent's stick away is not a preferred strategy, since it allows him to use the stick again. In most cases, it's better to take control of his stick.

Related Chapters:

- Attack
- The King of Strikes

STRIKE DRILLS

For the following drills, stand with your feet a little more than shoulder-width apart. Lead with your strong side and angle your body at 45° to your target. Point your feet toward your enemy.

The idea of this drill is to practice using circular forces. Roll your strikes using your waist. Most of your movement and power comes from your body motion, not your arm. Using only your arm and wrist limits your power. It's good for sport, to get fast points, but not very effective on the street. Big hits end fights.

These are primarily short-range strikes. Do not fully extend your arm when making them. You may get more distance, but will lose power at your shoulder. It will also make it easier for your opponent to manipulate your stick and/or grab arm.

Cutting Strikes

The strikes in this drill are considered long-range ones, and are good entry blows.

Aim to hit your target with the upper couple of inches of your stick. The strikes should go through your opponent in a cutting motion. Taken together, first four strikes form an infinity symbol.

Forehand to the head. From the starting position, bring your stick down diagonally across your body. Your opponent's temple and eye are your primary targets.

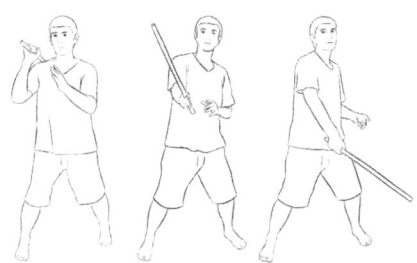

Backhand to the head. Bring the stick up your left side to the top of your left shoulder, then continue down diagonally across your body to your bottom right.

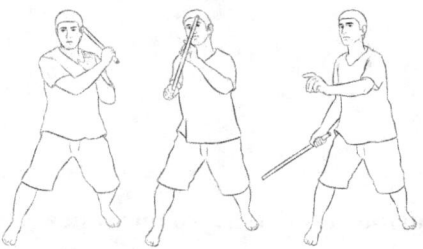

Forehand to the knee. Bring your stick up to shoulder height and squat down to lower your body. Strike down at your opponent's knee.

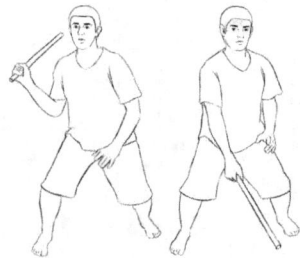

Backhand to the knee. Raise the stick up to your left shoulder. Stay low.

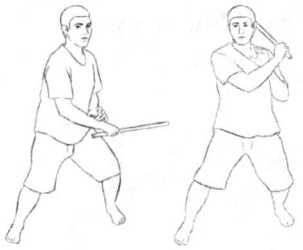

Do a backhand strike to your opponent's knee.

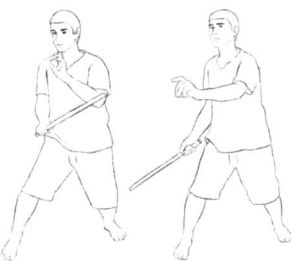

Repeat the previous four strikes a few times so you get used to using your waist.

Forehand Horizontal. After strike four, come back up and bring your stick back to waist height. Drive the stick horizontally to your left side. Your intention is to hit your opponent's elbow, wrist, or floating ribs if he has kept them open.

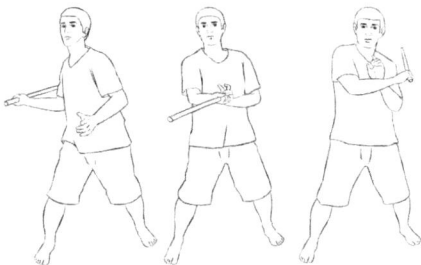

Backhand Horizontal. Move the stick back to your right side, more or less along the same path, but in reverse.

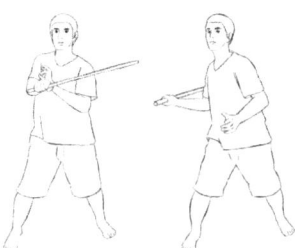

The King. Finish off with the king strike.

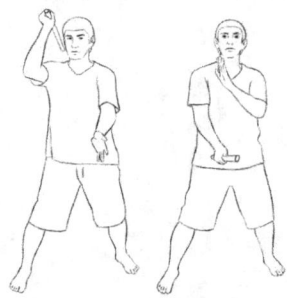

Bouncing Strikes

In this drill, you follow the same pattern as the cutting strikes drill, but the strikes are adapted for mid-range blows. At this range, you and your opponent are close enough to grab each other's weapons.

Bouncing strikes use a movement something between abanico and cutting strikes.

Contact is made from about halfway up the stick to the bottom of the top couple of inches.

Begin the first strike as before (forehand to the head). Instead of going through your opponent, your stick will make contact and then bounce off him.

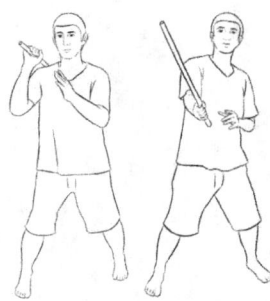

Using the momentum of the ricochet, guide your stick over your head in a circular abanico style and then make the second strike.

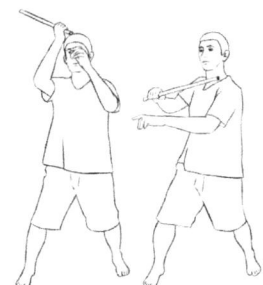

The same ricochet action is done for all seven of the strikes. Here are strikes three and four.

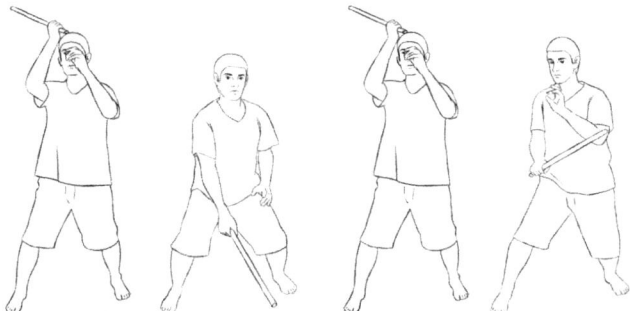

Strikes five and six.

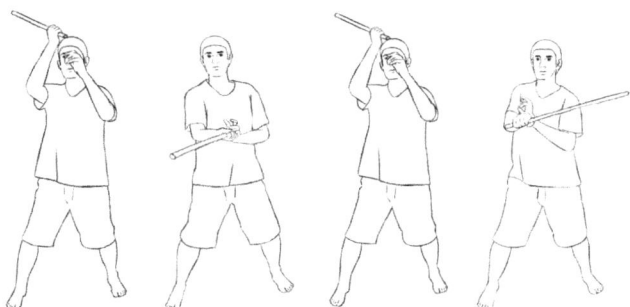

Strike seven.

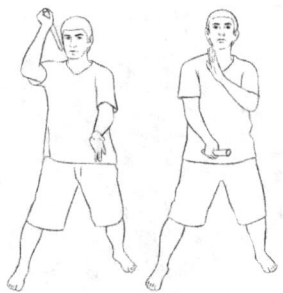

Rolling Strikes

This last set of strikes uses the same pattern again, but this time each strike is a double hit.

The double hit is achieved by rolling. Once the first strike crosses the center, you use your wrist to circle the strike over for a second hit before moving on to the next strike in the pattern. As an exercise, this move helps to develop flexibility, coordination, and strength in your wrist. In a fight, it is useful for making space, and/or as a way to exit if you think your opponent has had enough. Move back while doing it.

The number seven strike is not included in this drill.

The start of strike one is exactly the same as in the cutting strikes drill.

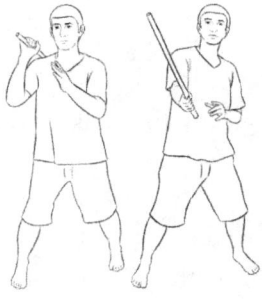

Once you cross center use your wrist to double up the strike and then continue to the other side.

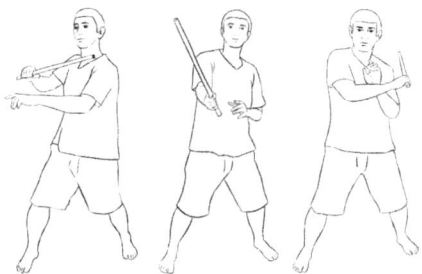

Strike two is the same as strike one, but backhand. Strikes three and four are the same as strikes one and two, respectively, except that they are aimed at your opponent's knee.

In strikes five and six, the double-up action is a circular movement over your head.

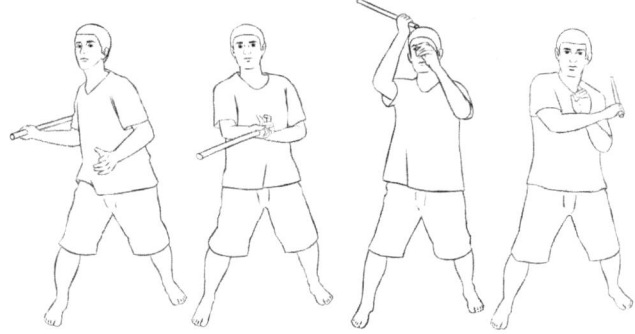

Strike Strategy

If you were to fight using only the strikes from these drills, the basic strategy would be to:

- Enter with cutting strikes.
- Batter your opponent with bouncing strikes.
- Exit with rolling strikes.

ABANICO DEFENSE

When both you and your opponent strike, but his timing is ahead of yours, you may choose to defend at the last instant. This defense works best when your opponent's strike is off center (not a pure seven). Both you and your opponent come in with overhead strikes. Your opponent's timing is just ahead of yours, so you quickly tap his weapon out of the way.

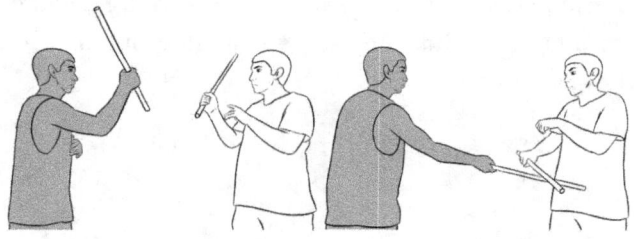

Use the abanico-style wrist flick coupled with the movement of your waist to renew your attack.

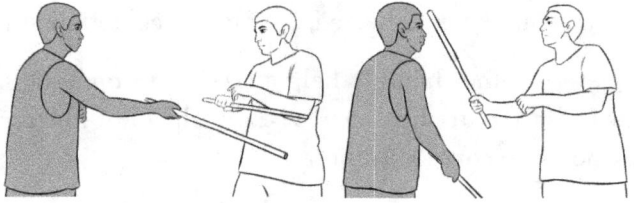

Whether you use a left or right tap depends on whether your opponent uses a number one or number two strike. You can close in as your opponent renews his attack.

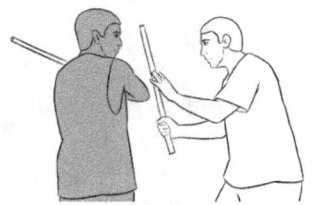

STICK PARRIES

When you are too close to use the abanico defense, stick parries are the answer. Deflect your opponent's attack (parry) and then counter with a strike or snatch.

If your opponent attacks with a number seven strike, you need to get off center to be able to parry it. To deflect on your right side, take a slightly angulated step forward and raise your hand a little so that your bent arm and stick form a triangle. This triangle will cause your opponent's attack to glide off. Do not angle your arm out. It will weaken the structure.

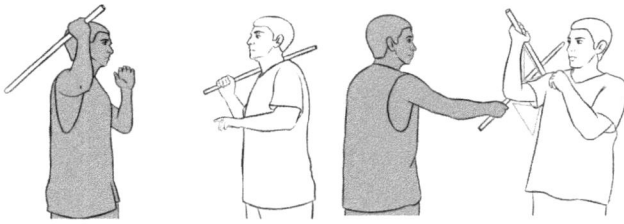

Once the attack has been deflected, counterattack (left picture below).

You can use your other hand to help guide your opponent's stick out of the way (right picture below). If you are ahead of his timing, your sticks may not even come into contact.

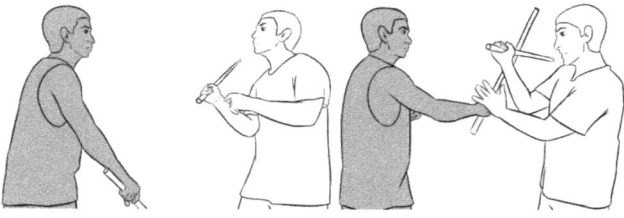

You may choose to go into a snatch. Here is one example.

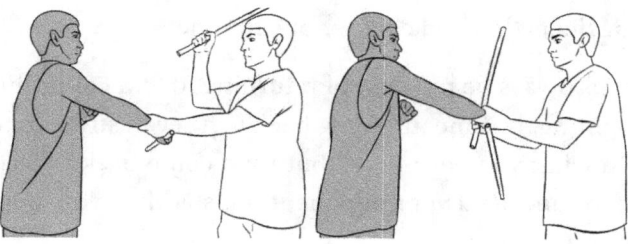

When you need to deflect on your left side, point your stick over your left shoulder. The triangle will be maintained.

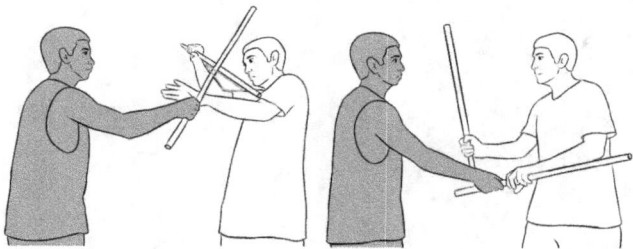

Returning to Seven

In this variation of the stick parries drill, you and your opponent alternate attack and defense positions. You do not grab each other's sticks. Your opponent strikes at you with a number seven. Parry and counter with your own number seven. As you counter, your opponent must bring his stick back to a seven. You will be quicker, so he will be obliged to concede and defend. Your opponent deflects your number seven and counters with his own number seven.

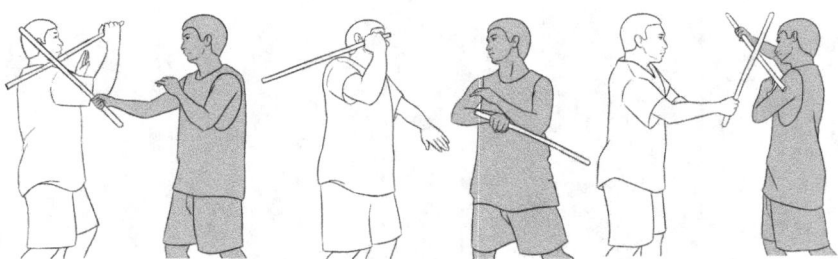

Repeat the deflection and counter one for one.

Important: Always be mindful of returning to and controlling center. In stick-fighting, this means going back to a seven strike (returning to seven). Do what you have to do, but then come back to a seven. You may have to concede if your opponent is faster than you, but return to the seven.

You can come in from the side if needed, but always aim to dominate the center, and once you are in, don't go back out.

Related Chapters:

- Attack
- Abanico Defense

DEFENSE DRILL

The previous two styles of defense (parry and abanico) can be practiced as a flow drill with a partner. Here is a sample progression.

1. Attacker strikes with alternating number one and two strikes. Defender defends using parries. Repeat this a few times.
2. Attacker strikes with alternating number one and two strikes. Defender defends using the abanico defense. Repeat this a few times.
3. Attacker strikes with number one and two strikes at his discretion. Defender uses parries, and can also counter when ready.
4. Attacker strikes with number one and two strikes at his discretion. Defender uses the abanico defense and can also counter when ready.

Related Chapters:

- Abanico Defense

SNATCHES

Snatching is when you take your opponent's stick from him. When you are fighting stick-on-stick, using the king strike is going to beat an average opponent 90% of the time.

When your opponent knows what he is doing, using a snatch is your next best option. This is because most stick systems don't involve grabbing the stick, so doing so gives you a major advantage.

All snatches begin with the seven defense. Once you've blocked your opponent's attack, use your free hand to take control of his weapon.

Note: For most snatches to work, you need to get your opponent's hand to your stick. When your hand touches your opponent's stick you can prevent a snatch by creating a small space (see Queen Defense and Counters) or by jumping (see Double-Grab Drill).

In the following demonstrations, all the attacks are either number one or number two strikes. However, with slight adjustments, the snatches can be applied to different strike angles. Even if your opponent uses a perfect king strike, you can turn it into an angled strike by blocking it on one side or the other.

Unless otherwise stated, in all these demonstrations you are the person on the right.

Snatch One: Stick on Stick

Your opponent attacks with a number one strike. Block the strike.

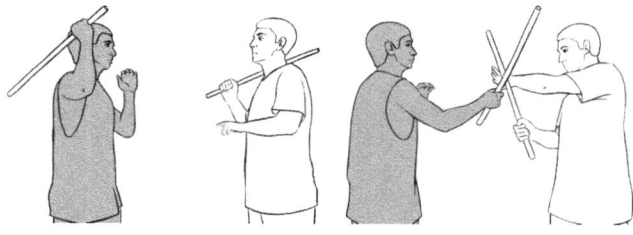

Grab the top of your opponent's stick with your left hand. Use an overhand grip (palm facing down).

Pull your opponent's stick down towards the outside of his guard, so that it's horizontal. The two sticks should form a cross, with your stick being close to your opponent's hand.

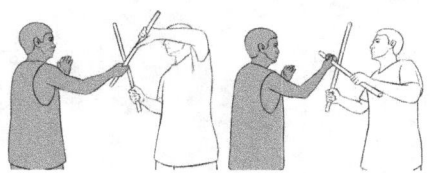

Push your opponent's stick into his face using a vortex motion, and then pry it out of his hand. Do so by using a waterfall action to push it past the outside of his shoulder. Finish with a butt strike (a strike with the bottom of your stick) to your opponent's face.

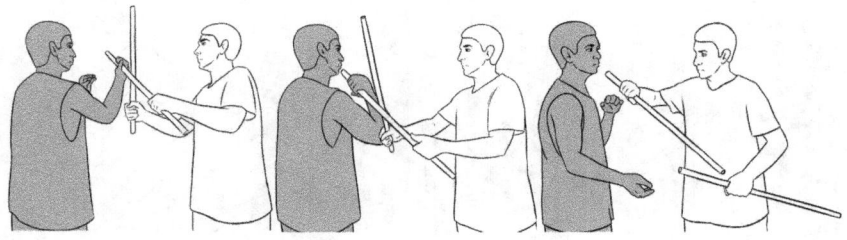

Snatch Two: Fist on Fist

Your opponent attacks with a number one strike. Block the strike.

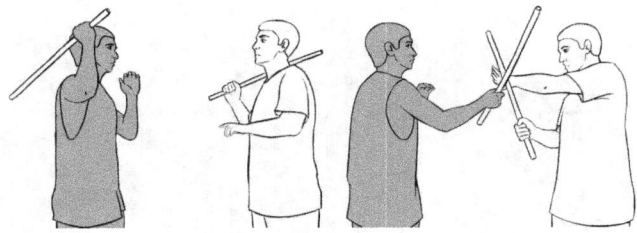

Grab the top of your opponent's stick with your left hand. Use an overhand grip.

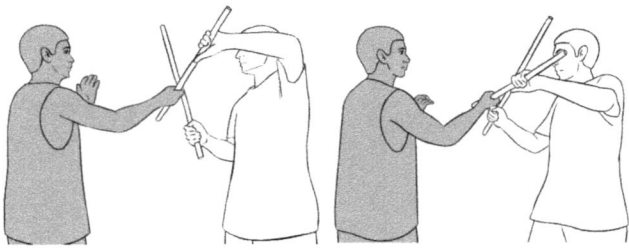

As you pull your opponent's stick down into the cross, place your right fist on the back of his right fist.

Push your opponent's stick into his face and then pry it out of his hand by pushing it past the outside of his shoulder.

Finish with a strike to your opponent's face.

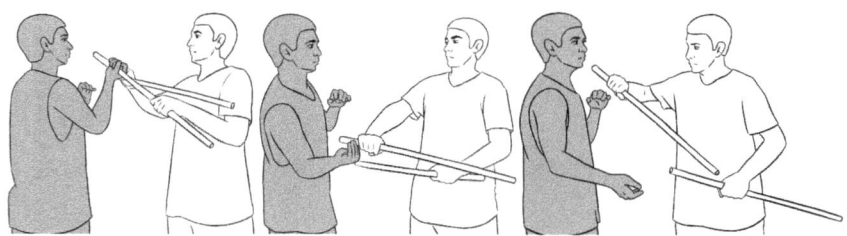

Snatch Three: Stick Lever

Your opponent attacks with a number one strike. Block the strike.

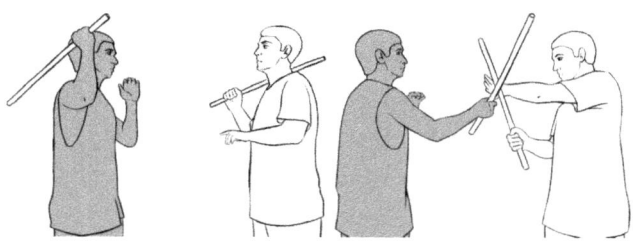

Grab the top of your opponent's stick with your left hand. Use an overhand grip.

Strike your opponent in the face with the butt of your stick, using a slight hooking motion.

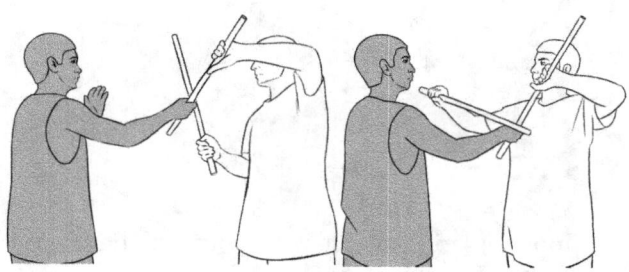

Continue along that path so that your right wrist lands on your opponent's right wrist. The end of your stick should be underneath your left armpit. Using your stick as a fulcrum, pry your opponent's stick out of his hand by pulling it down towards your left with your left hand.

You can thrust the butt of your stick into your opponent's face a few times if you need to.

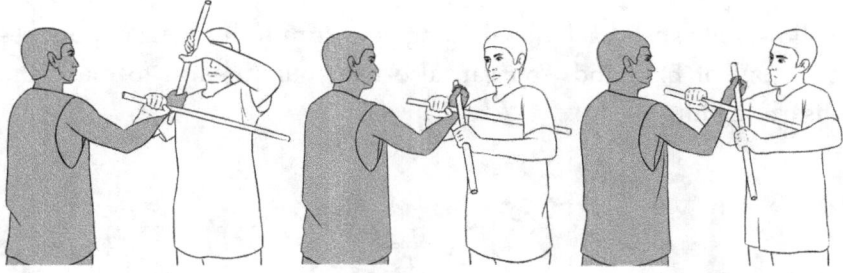

Snatch Four: Wrist Grab

Your opponent attacks with a number one strike. Block the strike.

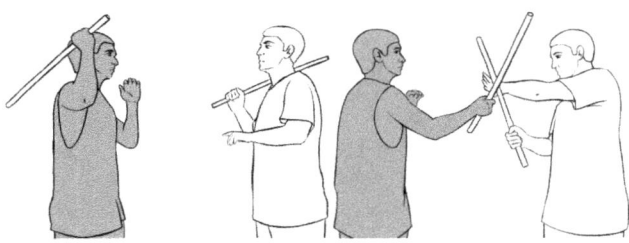

Grab your opponent's right wrist with your left hand and twist his arm slightly, so that his elbow faces the ground. Using your left arm as a guide, draw your stick back.

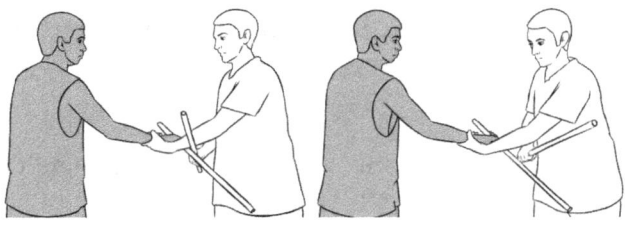

Follow your stick back down along your arm to hit your opponent's stick out of his hand. You can also use your forearm to make the disarming hit.

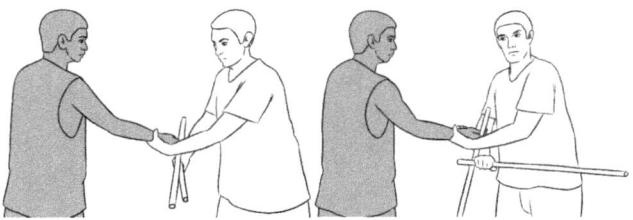

Snatch Five: Twist and Hit

Your opponent attacks with a number two strike. Block the strike.

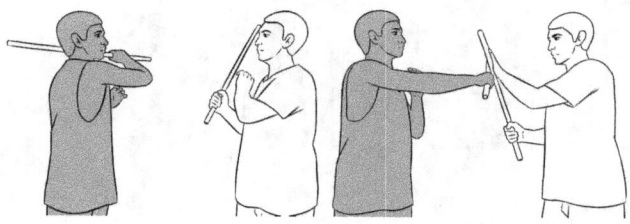

Grab your opponent's stick between his hand and your stick. Use an underhand grip (palm facing up).

Twist your opponent's stick down and continue to twist clockwise. This on its own may disarm him.

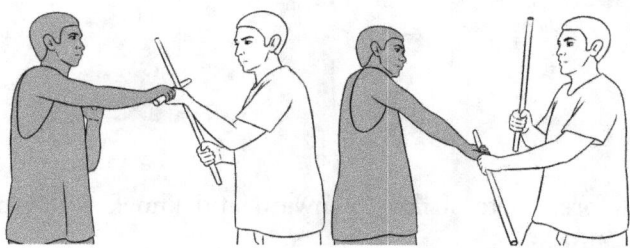

If not, use your lower left forearm (or the bottom of your stick) to strike his right wrist.

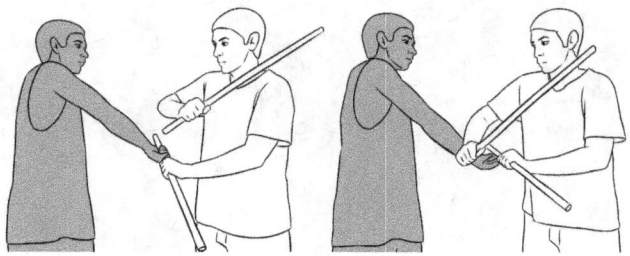

You can also use the back of your right elbow to strike the back of your opponent's right elbow.

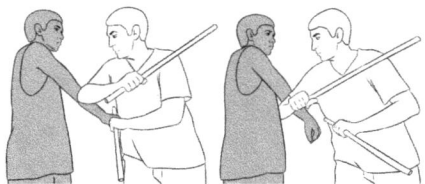

Snatch Six: But Strike

Your opponent attacks with a number two strike. Block the strike.

Grab your opponent's right wrist using an underhand grip.

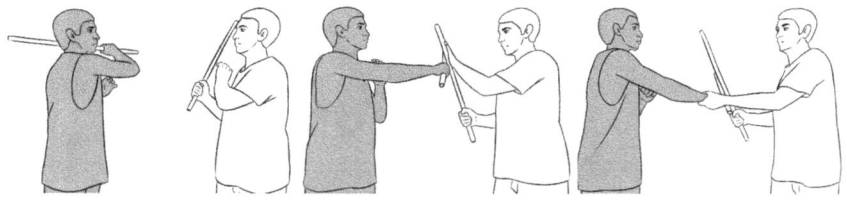

Use your forearm to strike downward and knock your opponent's stick out of his hand.

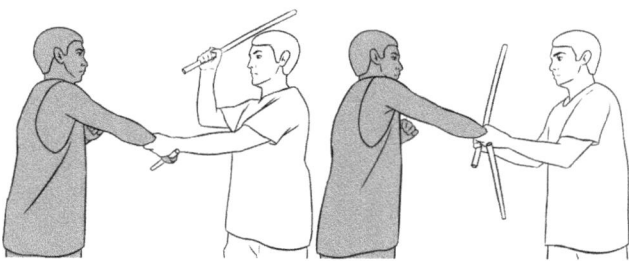

Snatch Seven: Twist and Pressure

Your opponent attacks with a number two strike. Block the strike.

Twist the bottom of your stick clockwise and over your opponent's stick. At the same time bring your left hand up underneath your opponent's right forearm.

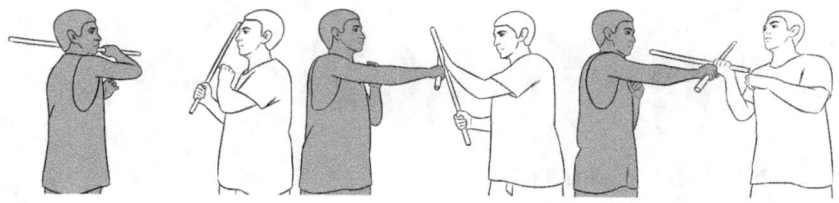

Apply downward pressure with your stick and upward pressure with your left hand to disarm your opponent.

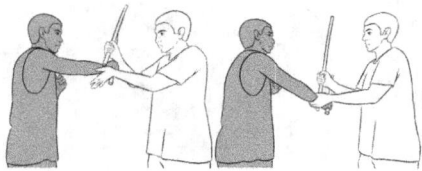

If this opposing pressure is not enough, draw your opponent's stick straight out towards you by pulling your stick back.

Hold your opponent's stick between your right arm and your body, and then use your left hand and a twist of your waist to push on the back of his right hand and move it to your right.

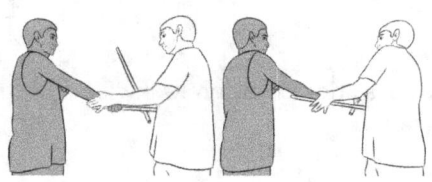

If that is still not enough, bring the bottom of your opponent's stick up and over his right hand. Twist back to your left and strike your opponent as you do so.

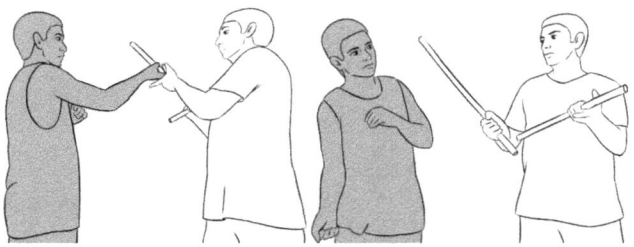

Snatch Eight: Hit and Twist

Your opponent attacks with a number two strike. Block the strike.

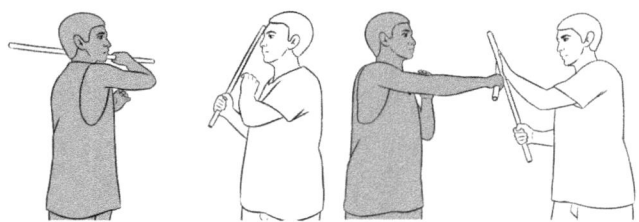

Grab your opponent's stick and push the top of it into his face.

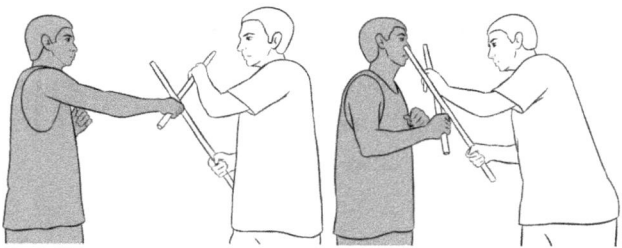

Twist your opponent's stick counterclockwise to your left, using your stick as a fulcrum.

As you do this, let the stick "spin" in your right hand, so that you finish with an overhand grip.

Once your opponent's stick is toward your left side, tighten your grip. Keep twisting until the stick comes out of your opponent's grip, and aim the bottom of it towards his groin. Not only will this hit him, it will also make it easier to get the stick out of his grip.

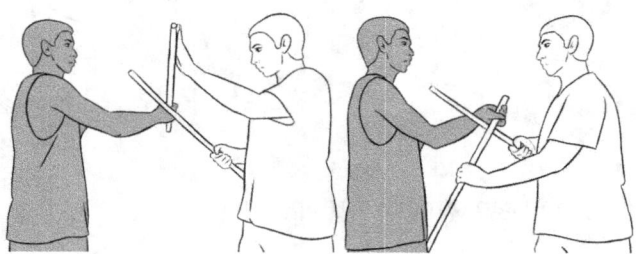

Snatch Nine: Arm Lever

Your opponent attacks with a number two strike. Block the strike.

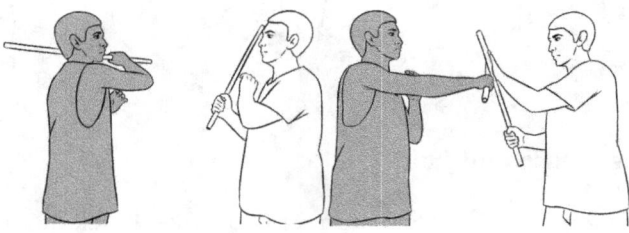

Grab your opponent's stick and then lower it, so you can thrust the tip of your stick into him.

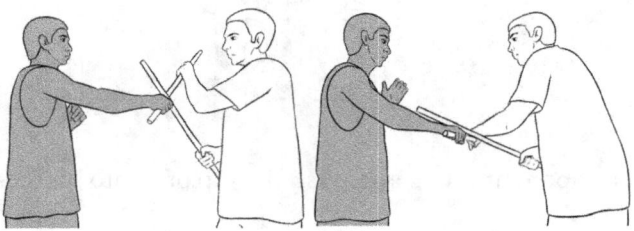

Do a second thrust past your opponent's head (or if you missed the first one) and then use your arm as the fulcrum point to disarm your opponent, in the same way as in snatch eight.

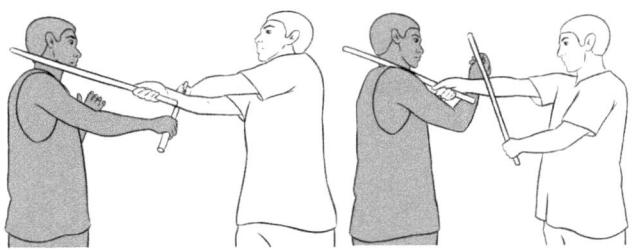

Alternatively, you can punch your opponent.

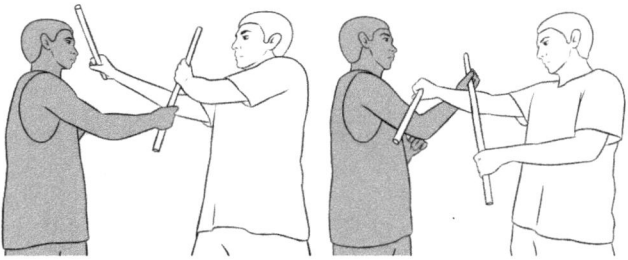

Snatch Ten: Push and Pull

Your opponent attacks with a number two strike. Block the strike.

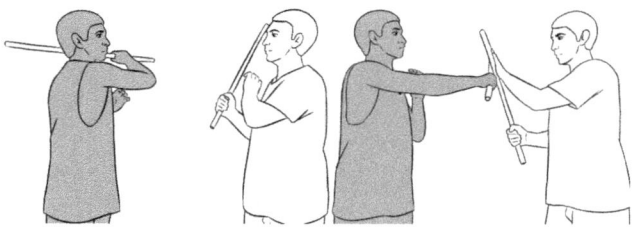

Grab your opponent's stick and push the top of it into his face.

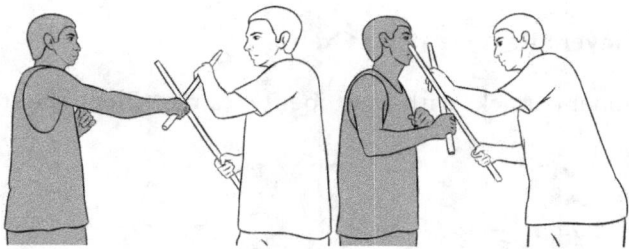

Change your grip so that your palm faces your left, and then pull your opponent's stick back towards you so that his hand is up against your stick.

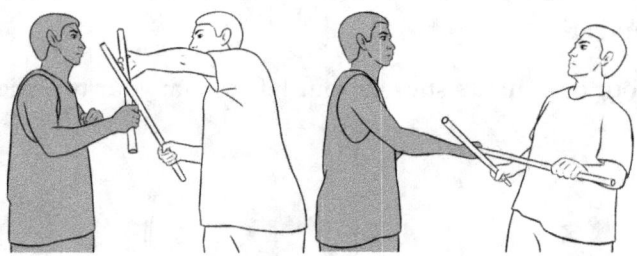

Push towards your opponent to make his arm collapse, and then pull back to take the stick.

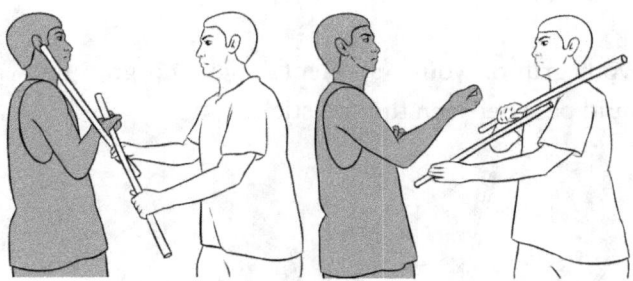

Snatch Eleven: Reverse Wrist Grab

Your opponent attacks with a number two strike. Block the strike.

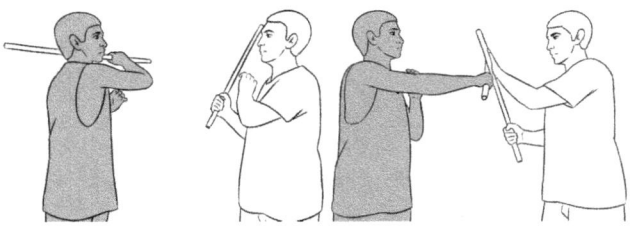

Grab your opponent's stick between your stick and his hand. Use an underhand grip.

Rotate your opponent's stick to your left so that your two sticks make a cross.

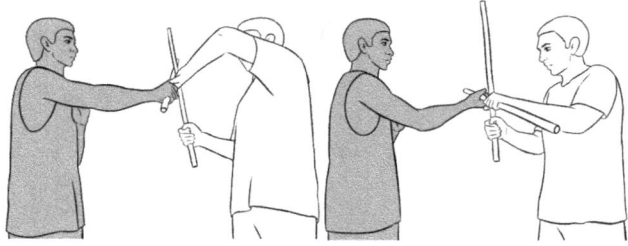

Release your grip on your opponent's stick and grab his wrist. Your hand should pass between the two sticks.

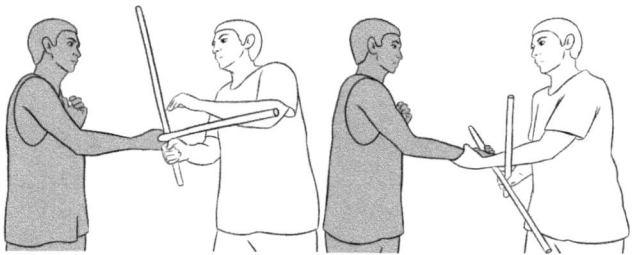

Use your forearm to knock the stick out of your opponent's hand.

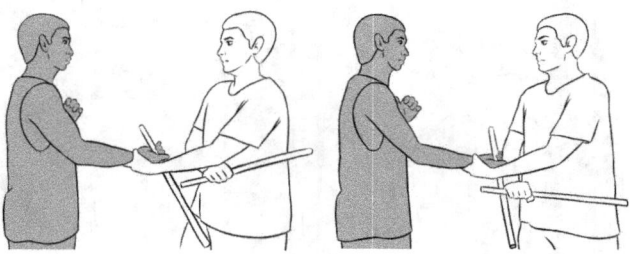

Snatch Twelve: Weave and Pull

Your opponent attacks with a number two strike. Block the strike.

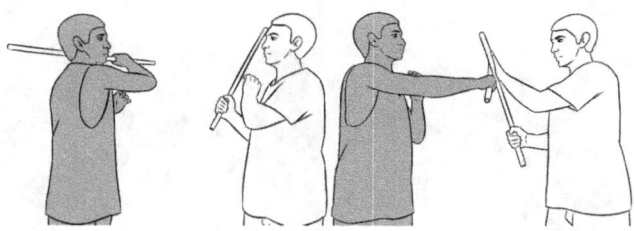

Weave your hand over your opponent's stick between your stick and his hand and then under your opponent's wrist to your left.

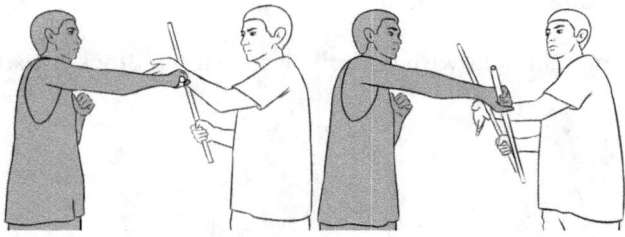

Maneuver your stick so it is positioned horizontally over your opponent's forearm and then grab the end of it with your left hand.

Pull towards yourself to dislodge your opponent's stick.

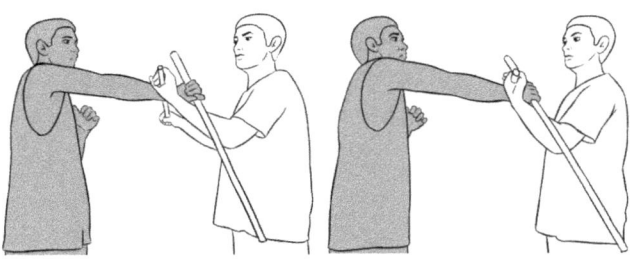

The same weaving maneuver can be used on your opponent's upper arm. Apply a painful lock with downward pressure. You can then slide your stick back to your opponent's wrist to disarm him as before.

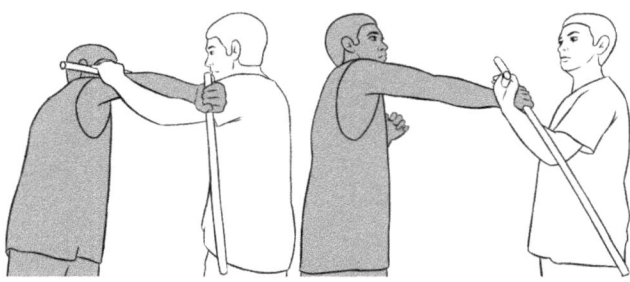

Snatch Thirteen: Wrist Slam

Your opponent attacks with a number two strike. Block the strike.

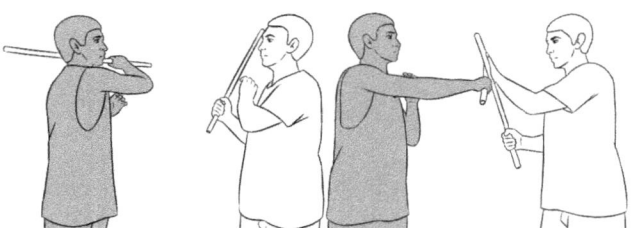

Grab your opponent's stick and lower it so you can thrust the tip of your stick into him.

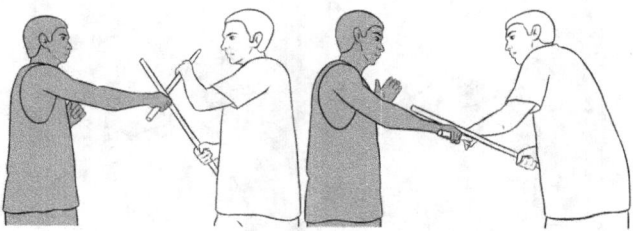

Pass your stick under your opponent's arm and toward your left side. As you do this, quickly put your right hand on top of his hand.

Maneuver the bottom of your stick so it is on top of your opponent's lower arm.

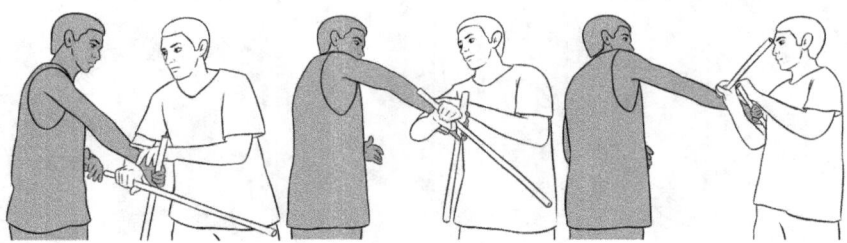

Use your left hand to slam down on your stick where it is on your opponent's arm.

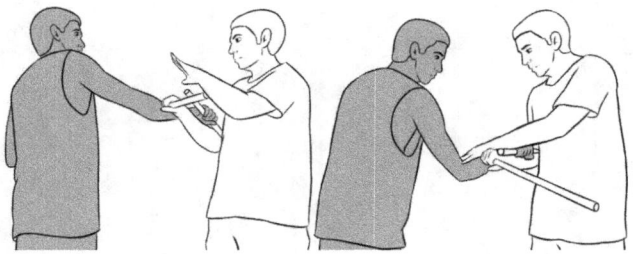

An alternative to slamming down on your stick is to push the top of your stick into your opponent's head.

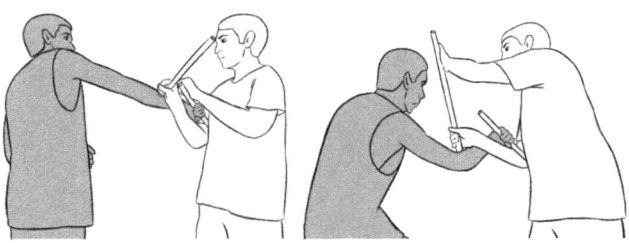

Related Chapters:

- The King of Strikes
- Queen Strike
- Double-Grab Scenarios

GRAB AND STRIKE DRILLS

In the snatches chapter, you learned how stick grabbing enables you to take your opponent's weapon. In the exercises in this chapter, you'll be grabbing your opponent's stick and then moving it out of the way so you can strike him.

This chapter also delves into advanced strikes. In this demonstration, you are in the position of the person on the right in the pictures.

This is all one drill, but has been split into three parts—basic, intermediate, advanced—for ease of learning.

Basic Grab and Strike Drill

This drill makes use of the seven cutting strikes as well as a modified queen strike.

Your opponent strikes with a number seven hit. Defend with a number seven so that the top of your opponent's stick will be inside your guard.

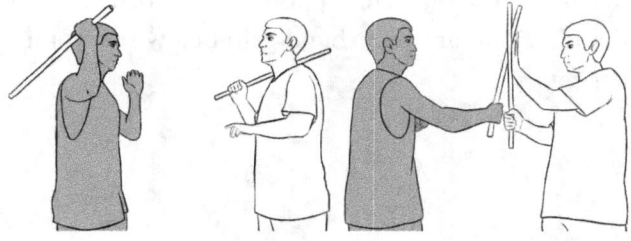

Grab his stick with your left hand using an overhand grip above the point where the two sticks meet.

Prepare to strike by pulling his stick to the left side of your head while bringing your stick to the outside of your left side.

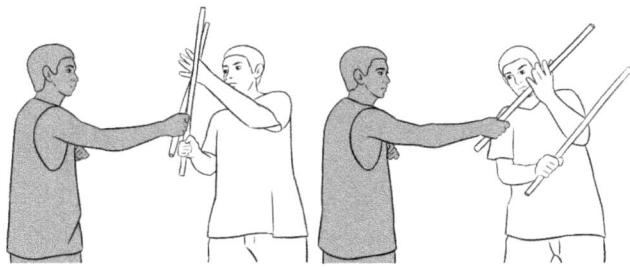

Strike with a number four hit to his knee.

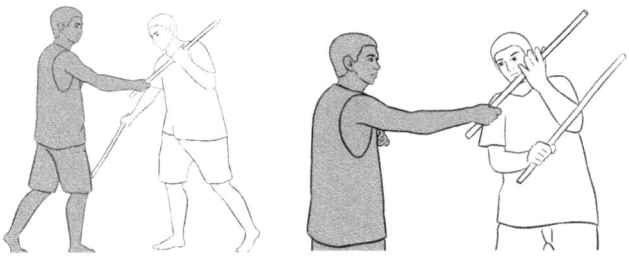

Place your stick back on your opponent's to form a cross. Change your left-hand grip to an underhand grip below the point where the two sticks meet.

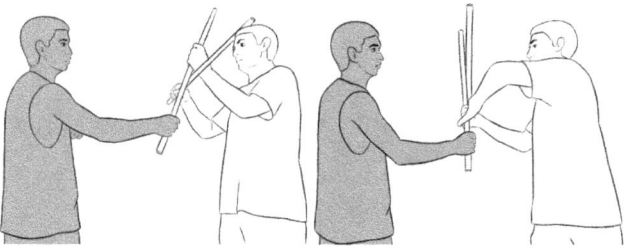

Hit his lead knee using a number three strike.

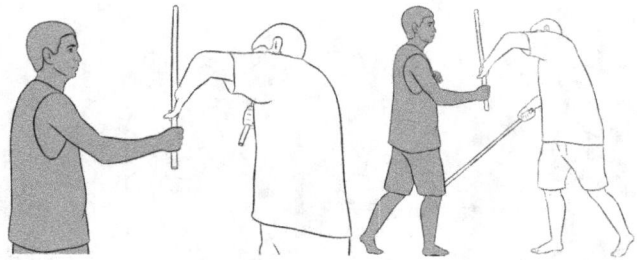

Place your stick back on his to form a cross.

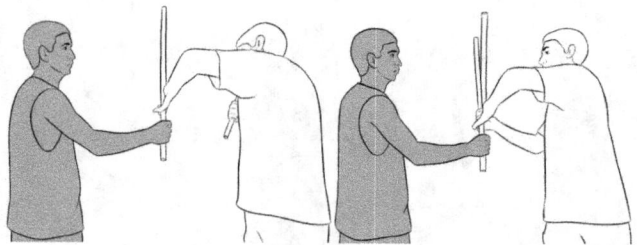

Prepare for your next strike by pulling his stick down to your left side and over your left shoulder, then strike with a number two hit.

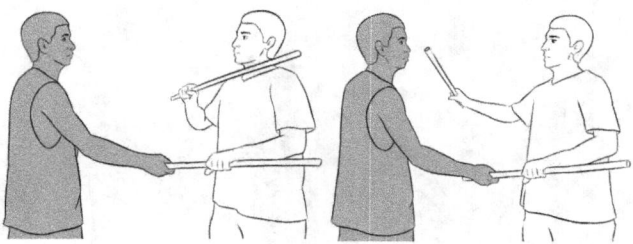

Pull your stick back over your left shoulder. Place your stick back on your opponent's to form a cross.

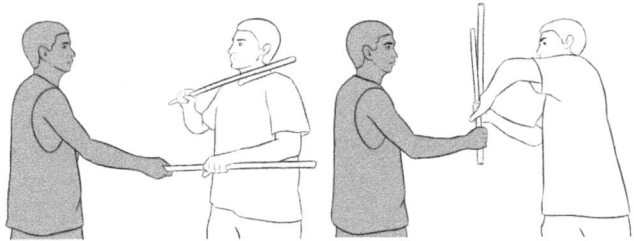

Change your left hand to an overhand grip below the point where the two sticks meet and then pull your opponent's stick down and to your right.

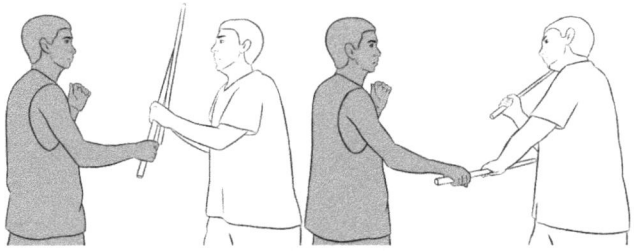

Strike with a number one hit.

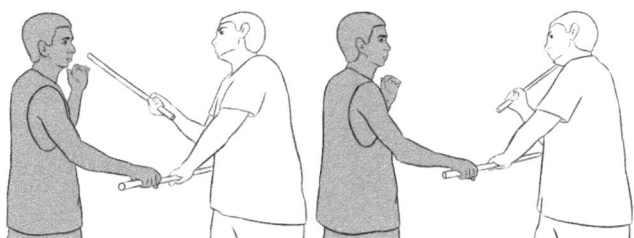

Place your stick back on your opponent's to form a cross, and then move your left hand above the point where the two sticks meet. Use an overhand grip.

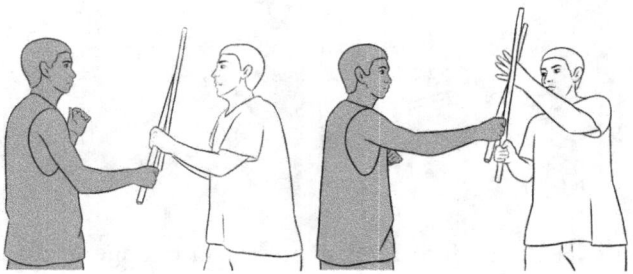

Lower his stick a bit and then use a queen strike to hit his face. Your strike should go over his stick.

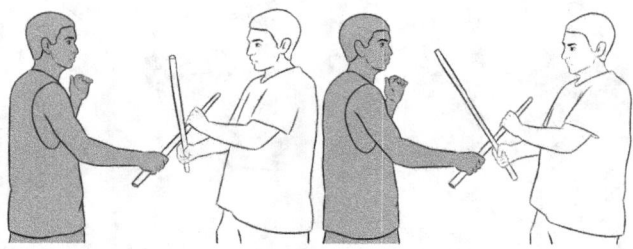

Change your left-hand grip to an underhand grip below the point where the two sticks meet and then pull your opponent's stick to your left as you pull yours to your right.

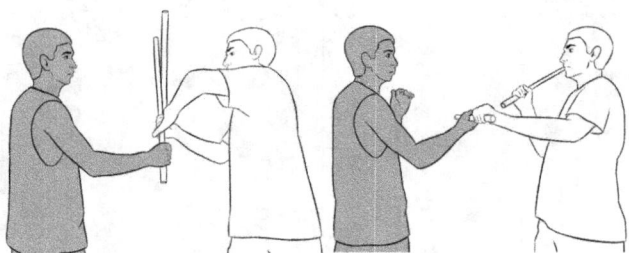

Strike your opponent with a number one strike and then pull your stick back and to your right.

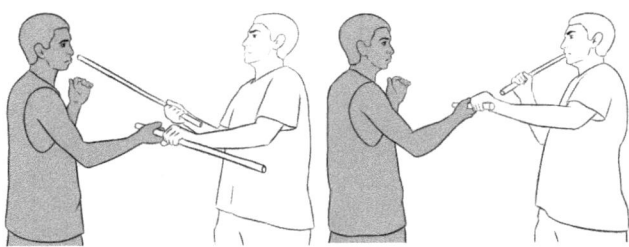

Bring the sticks back into a cross and then change to an overhand grip.

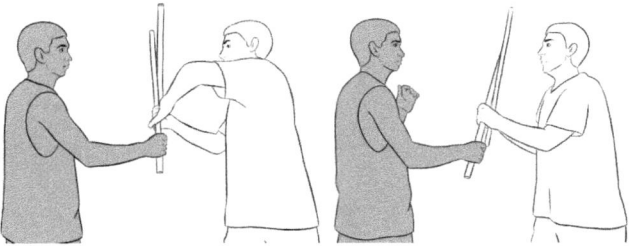

Push your opponent's stick down and to your right, then strike with a number seven hit.

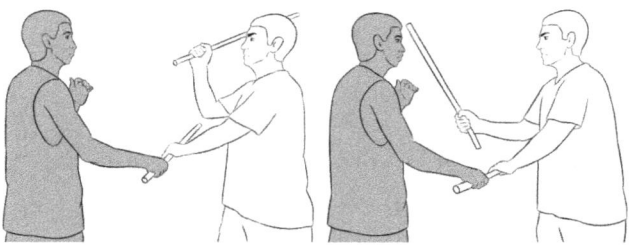

Bring the sticks back into a cross.

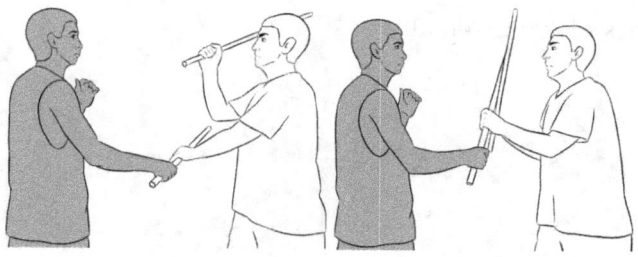

Intermediate Grab and Strike Drill

Rolling and abanico strikes are used in this stage of the drill.

Start in the finishing position from the basic grab and strike drill, sticks in a cross.

Push your opponent's stick down and strike with a rolling number seven strike.

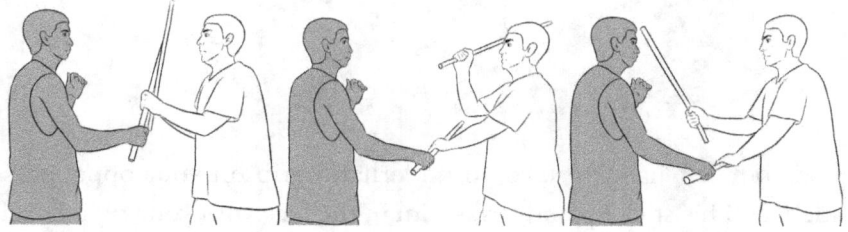

The rolling strike should travel down the outside of your opponent's right side.

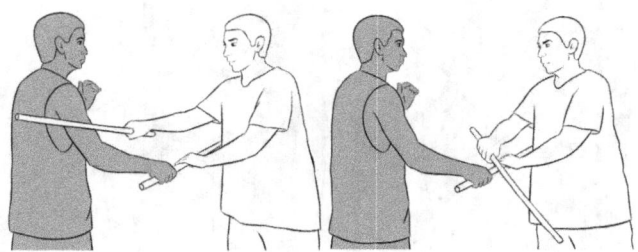

It should then continue on a circular path, coming up on the outside of your left shoulder and down, so that your stick crosses on your opponent's stick horizontally.

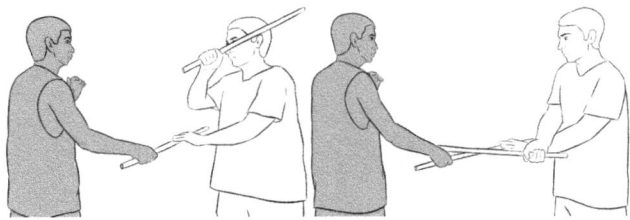

Step to the outside of your opponent's guard. Use your left hand to cover your opponent's right forearm and then strike him in the face, either with your fist or with the bottom of your stick.

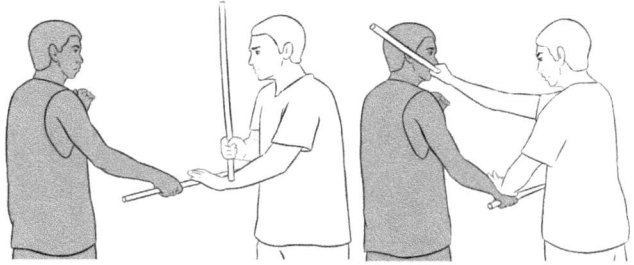

Use your left hand to take an underhand grip on your opponent's stick. Pull his stick up and strike him in the face with your right hand (or stick). At the same time, change to an overhand grip with your left hand.

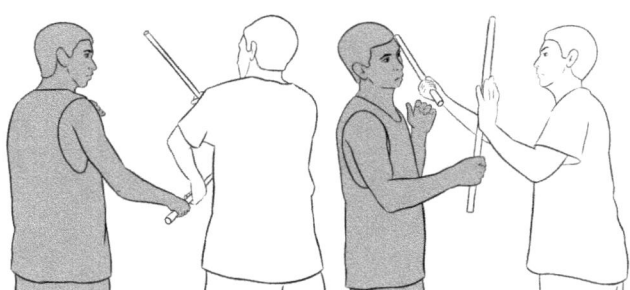

Push your opponent's stick back down and do an abanico hit to the right side of his head.

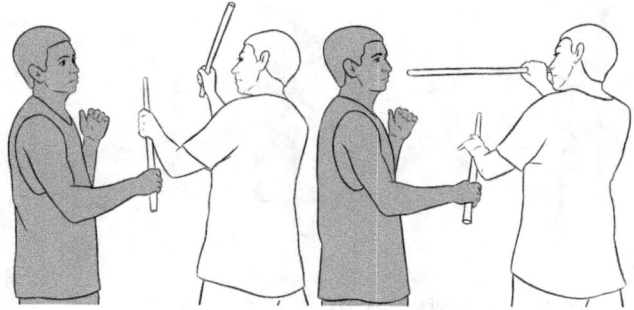

Rotate your stick in the opposite direction to ma an abanico hit to the left side of your opponent's head. Whilst rotating your stick, hit your opponent in the face with his own stick.

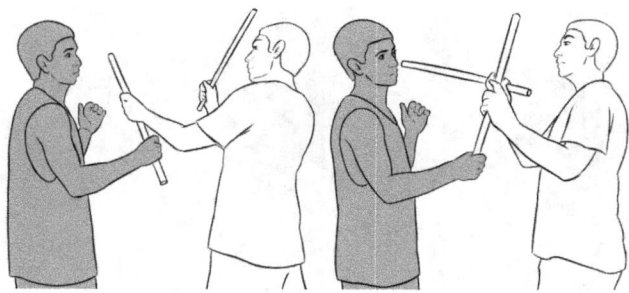

Return your stick to a number seven position and continue through with a rolling hit.

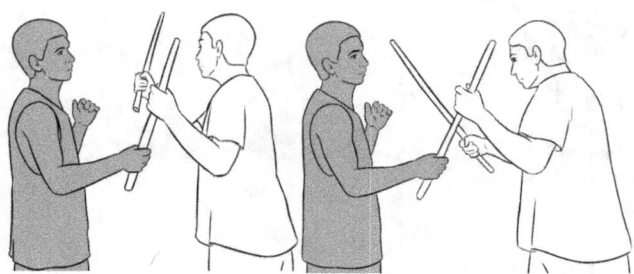

This hit should finish with you holding your stick at waist height, pointing it towards your opponent.

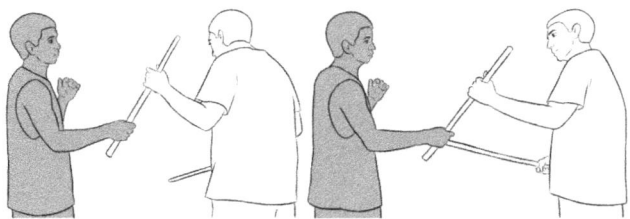

Advanced Grab and Strike Drill

This final stage of the grab and strike drill uses slashing and stabbing strikes. Start by hitting your opponent with the top of his own stick as you bring your stick back up to your right shoulder.

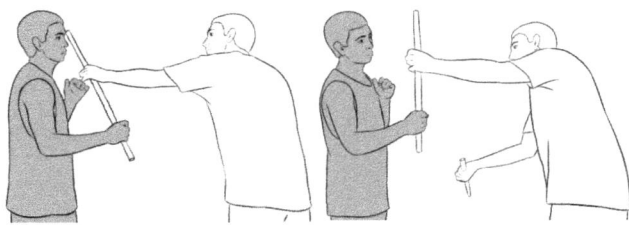

Do a number three strike which slashes through him and ends at your left hip.

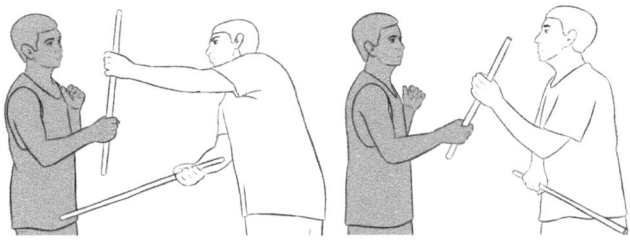

Hit your opponent with the top of his own stick and then do a number four strike through him.

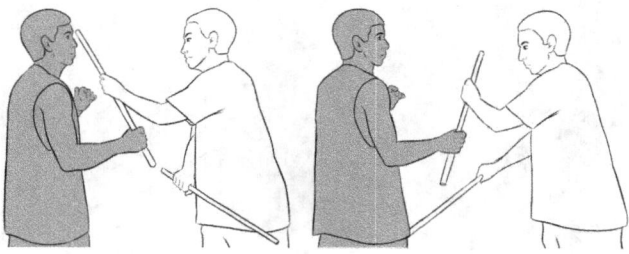

Finish the strike at your right hip and then pull your opponent's stick down.

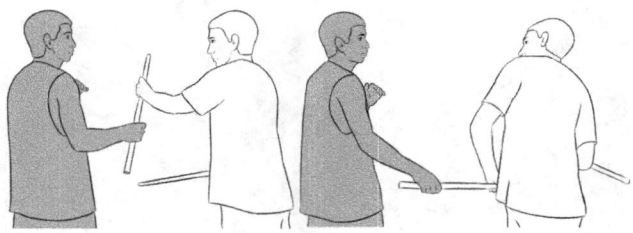

Do an upwards slashing strike through his head, from bottom right to top left. The tip of your stick should end up behind your left shoulder.

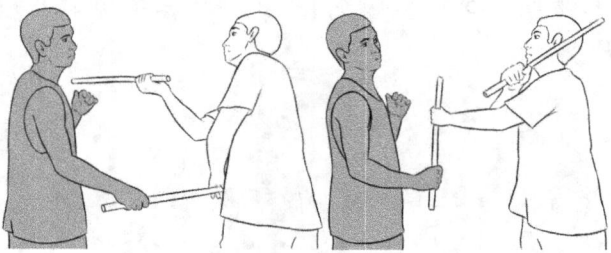

Hit your opponent with the top of his own stick and then pull it down to your left.

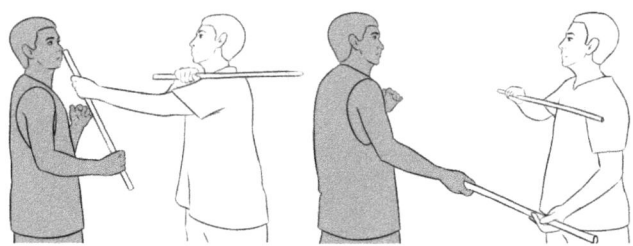

Do a horizontal back-hand strike through your opponent's head and quickly follow up by hitting him with the top of his own stick in a semi-circular motion from (your opponent's) right to left.

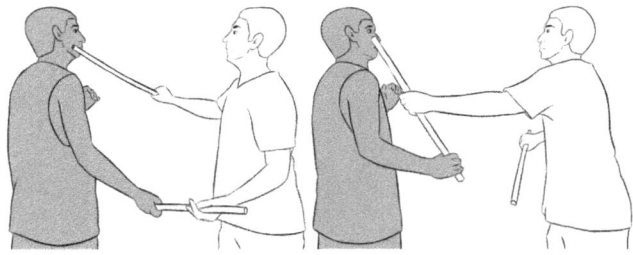

As you complete this strike, bring the tip of your stick near your left hip.

Use a queen strike to hit your opponent's face. Your strike should go over his stick.

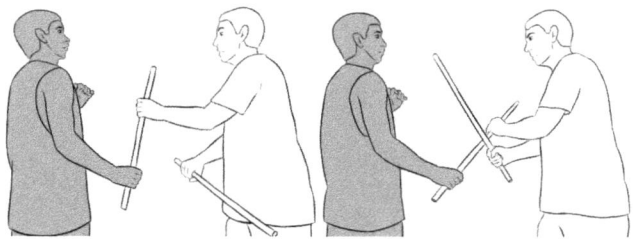

Use another queen strike to hit your opponent's stick away.

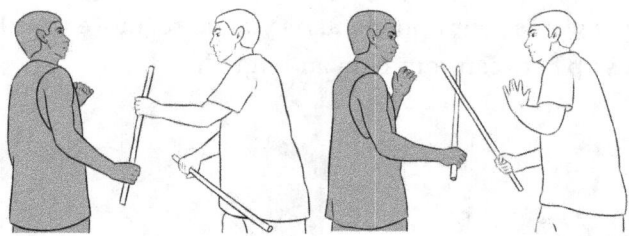

As you do so, quickly cover his right hand with your left and then use a hooking motion from (your) right to left to drive the tip of your stick through your opponent's face.

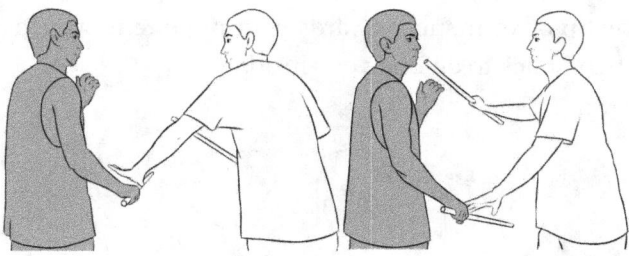

Continue to thrust your stick past your opponent's face.

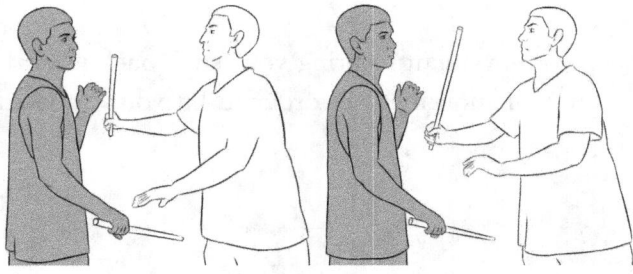

Once the tip of your stick is past your opponent's face, bring your right hand to your own upper left side while turning the tip of your stick back towards your opponent. As you do so, move your left hand also comes up between your chin and right hand.

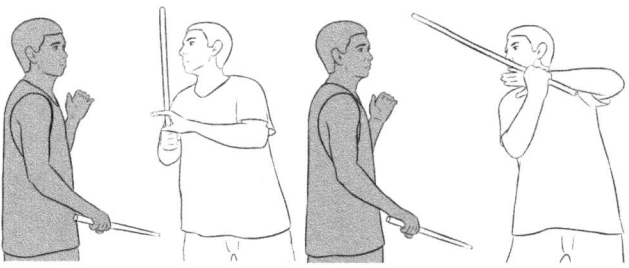

Thrust the tip of your stick towards your opponent's face as you pull your left hand back to defend your head.

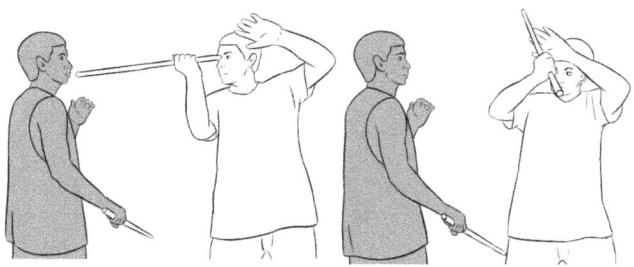

Use an abanico movement to bring your stick back toward you and down in a circular movement in order to hit your opponent in the groin.

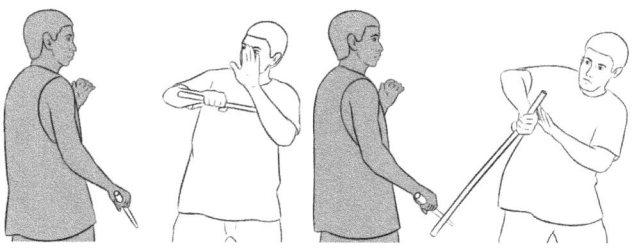

Let your stick bounce back and over.

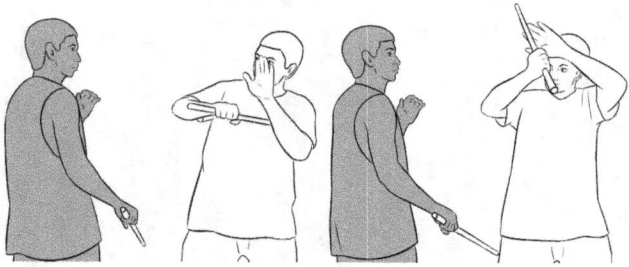

Use the momentum to hit your opponent in the top of the head.

Start to step back with your right foot as you bring your stick up and out.

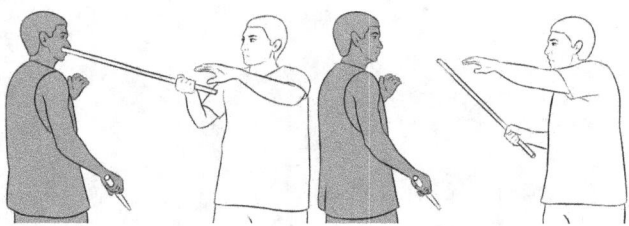

Strike your opponent with the tip of your stick using a right overhand thrust.

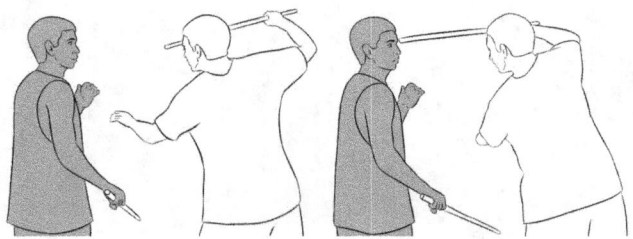

This completes the full grab and strike drill.

Related Chapters:

- Queen Strike
- Snatches

GRAB AND STRIKE DEFENSE DRILLS

Grab and Strike Defense Drill One

This flow drill shows how to defend against someone who grabs your stick and strikes. It demonstrates defense against the first four strikes from the previous chapter (grab and strike) which you can then adapt to any strike. It also contains a few examples (of the many that are possible) of snatch opportunities along the way.

In this demonstration, you take the position of the person on the right in the pictures. The person on the left is doing the grab and strike drill from the previous chapter and you are defending against his strikes. Strike at your opponent with a number seven hit. Your opponent defends with a number seven so that the top of your stick will end up inside his guard.

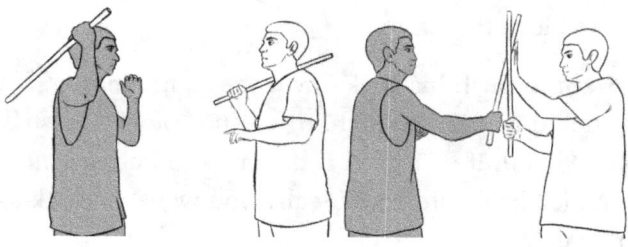

Your opponent grabs your stick with his left hand using an overhand grip above the point where the two sticks meet. He pulls back to strike you with a number four hit.

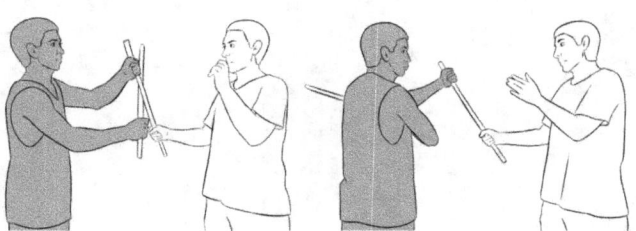

As your opponent strikes, use your left hand to block his right hand.

At the same time, pull the bottom of your stick down so that his stick hits it between your right and his left hand. Return to the cross position.

Your opponent switches his left-hand grip to an underhand grip below the point where the two sticks meet.

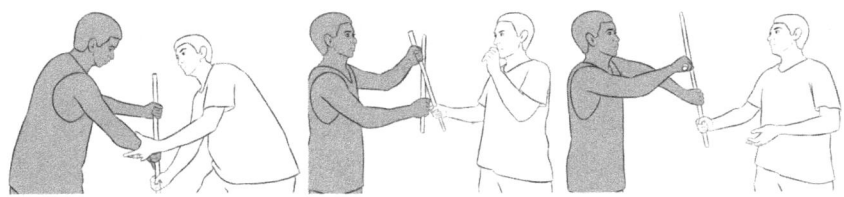

Your opponent pulls back to strike with a number three hit.

As the strike comes in, use your left hand to hit down on your opponent's left wrist from the outside of his guard. This will move your stick down to block the strike.

It is important to push his stick down the right amount. If you don't push the stick down far enough, it will not block the strike, and it may hit your hand. If you push it down too much, it will knock the top of your stick back into you. Ideally, you want the stick to hit your opponent's hand.

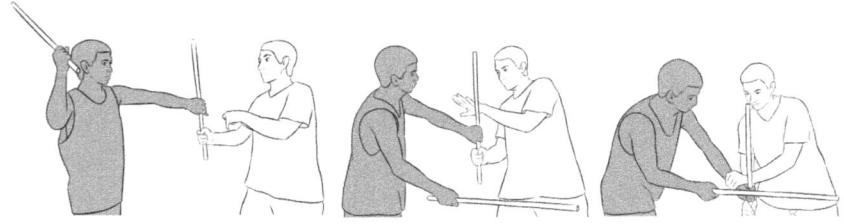

From this position you can do a queen strike. This is not part of the drill.

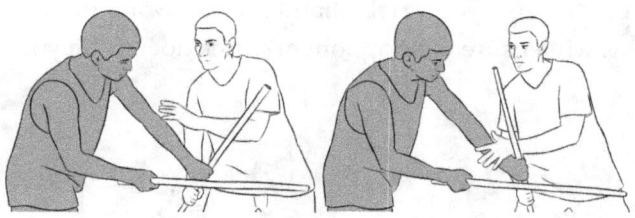

Training Tip: Practice these first movements until you're proficient before moving on.

You both return to the cross position, and then your opponent pulls your stick down and to your right as he pulls back for a number two strike.

As the strike comes in, simultaneously raise the bottom of your stick and use your left hand to hit down on your opponent's stick. This will ensure your opponent's stick doesn't hit your hand.

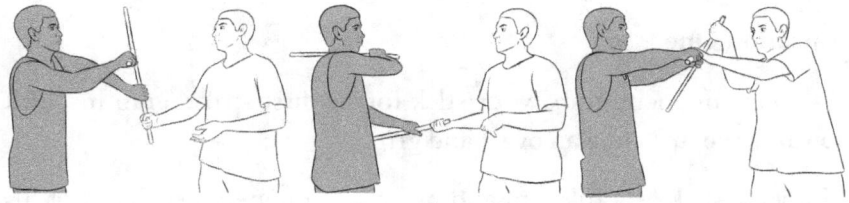

Return to the cross position. Your opponent changes to a forward grip. Your opponent pulls your stick down and to his right as he pulls back for a number one hit.

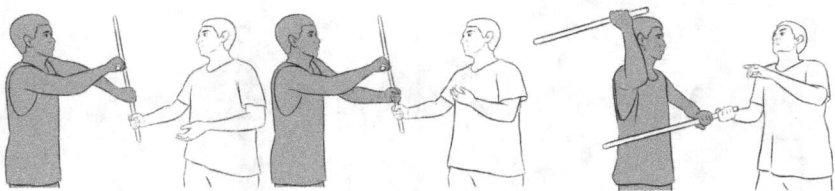

As the strike comes in, turn your body to the left and bend at your knees as you raise the bottom of your stick to protect your head.

If you need to, use your right hand to pull your opponent's stick down. This will ensure your opponent's stick doesn't hit your hand.

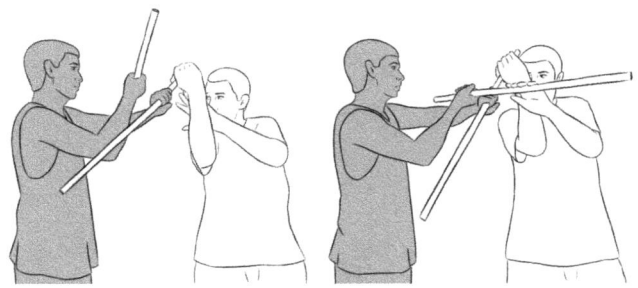

Throughout the whole Grab and Strike Defense Drill, there are opportunities to strike, snatch, etc. The following examples outline small fraction of the possibilities to give you an idea of what can be done. Once you're proficient at the drill, progress to adding additional attacks.

Variation One

As your opponent grabs your stick for his first strike, grab his stick towards the tip, using an overhand grip.

Use your stick as a fulcrum and pry your opponent's stick out of his hand by circling it counterclockwise. As you do the circling movement, allow your opponent's stick to spin in your palm and/or fingers, so that you're able to smoothly change grip as needed.

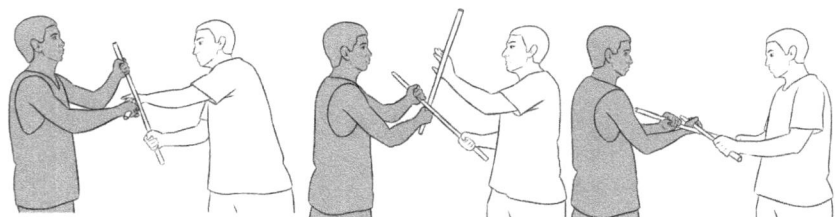

Variation Two

As your opponent grabs your stick for his first strike, grab his stick at a point between his hand and your stick using an underhand grip.

Circle the stick clockwise until your opponent's palm faces up. Use your right hand to strike downward on your opponent's wrist and disarm him.

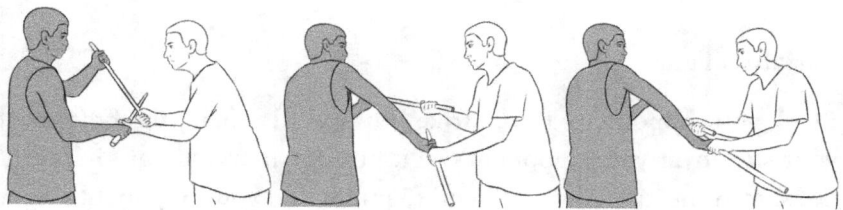

Variation Three

If you were unable to rotate the stick clockwise, as in example two (perhaps your opponent's grip was too strong), reverse your grip. That is, use an underhand grip, but with your elbow pointing up.

Rotate your opponent's stick counterclockwise and place your right fist on the back of his right fist.

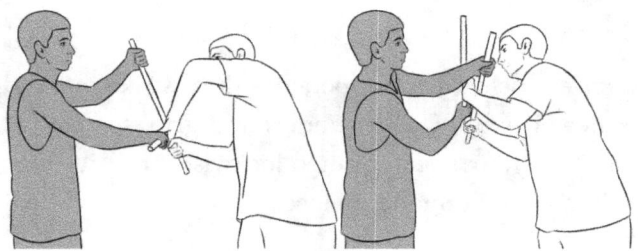

Push your opponent's hand towards his face. This will tangle him up. Continue to push.

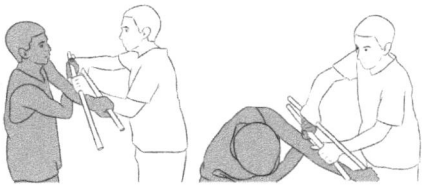

Variation Four

Block your opponent's third strike in the drill. Rotate the bottom of your stick over your opponent's so it hits down on his right hand. At the same time, use your left hand to pull up on your opponent's right hand.

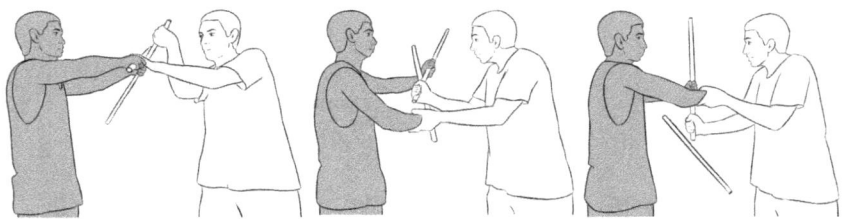

Variation Five

After you have blocked your opponent's third strike in the drill, grab your stick near the tip. Use an underhand grip, so that your elbow faces up. Rotate your stick counterclockwise until it's vertical, and then push it into your opponent's face.

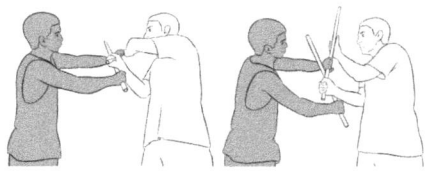

Variation Six

Block your opponent's fourth strike in the drill and then, from the defensive position, use your stick as a fulcrum and pry your opponent's stick out of his hand.

You can also push your opponent's stick into his head.

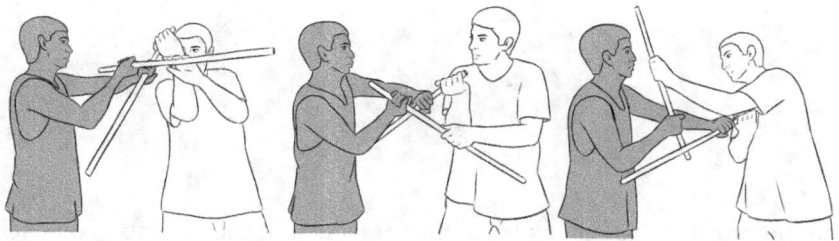

Grab and Strike Defense Drill Two

This drill is the same as the grab and strike defense drill, except the defender is more proactive. He hits the attacker's hand off his (the defender's) stick and then counterattacks.

In the following examples, you are the person on the left.

As your opponent does the first strike in the drill (a number four), use your left hand to block his right hand. At the same time, pull the bottom of your stick down, so that your opponent's stick hits it between your right and his left hand.

Use your left hand to slap his left hand off your stick.

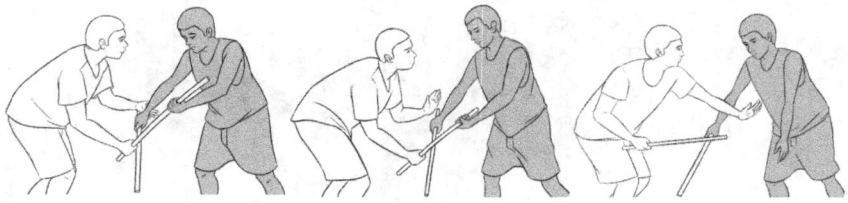

Continue with the grab and strike defense as normal.

As your opponent does the second strike (a number three), use your left hand to block his right hand. At the same time, pull the bottom of your stick down, so that your opponent's stick hits it between your right and his left hand. Use your left hand to slap his left hand off your stick.

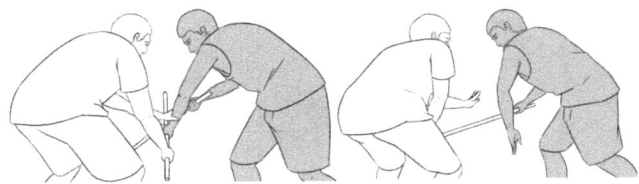

As his third strike comes in, deflect it as usual, then bring your stick back over into a king strike.

Deflect the final strike as usual.

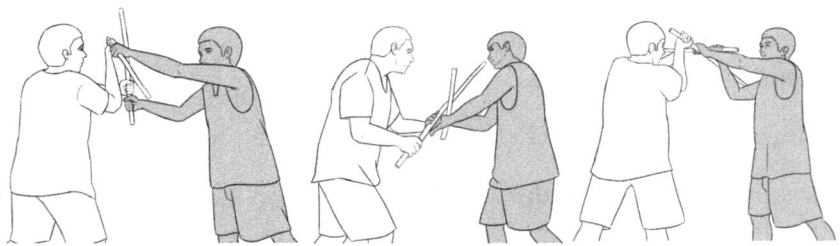

Then bring your stick back over into a king strike.

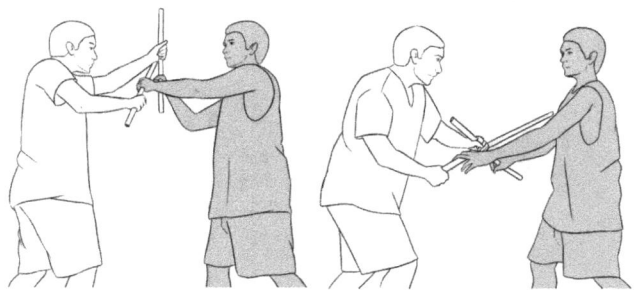

Grab and Strike Defense Drill Three

In this drill, you practice getting your opponent's stick and using it against him, and as in the previous drill, you also practice going back to seven (the king strike).

It's better to hit your opponent with his stick than your hand. It will hurt him more and give you control of his stick.

To increase his pain, aim for bony areas, rather than muscle, when striking your opponent with his stick as opposed to muscle.

From the first defensive position, use your right hand to grab your opponent's stick in the space between your stick and his right hand.

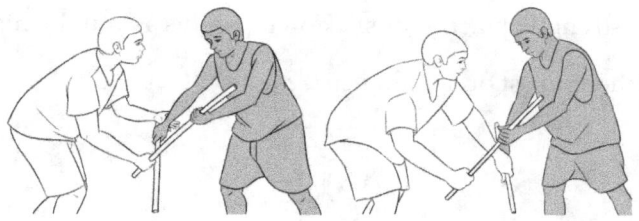

Use his stick to hit his arm from below. Adopt the seven position and then continue to the second defensive position.

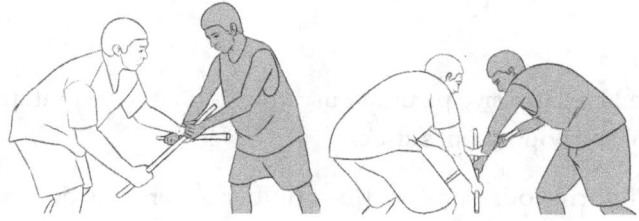

Grab the upper section of your opponent's stick and bring it up and over to hit his left arm. At the same time, place your stick on top of his to come into the seven position.

This will also give you more leverage when you're hitting him with his own stick.

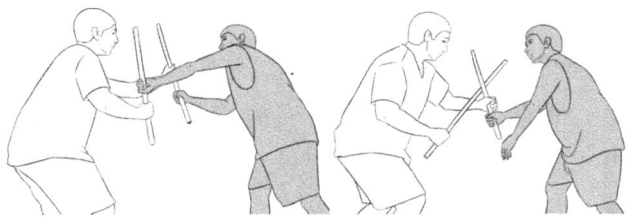

As you adopt the third defensive position, swing your stick into the number seven position and use his stick to hit his left arm from above.

For extra strength, place your stick on top of his as you do this.

You can then thrust or do other strikes.

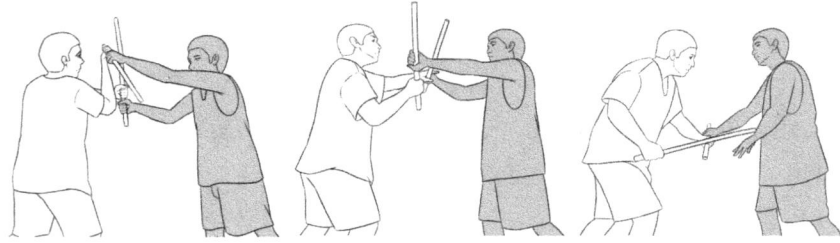

From the last defensive position, use your left hand to grab the upper section of your opponent's stick.

As you return your stick to the number seven position, use your opponent's stick to strike down on his left arm. For extra strength, place your stick on top of his as you do this. You can then thrust or do other strikes.

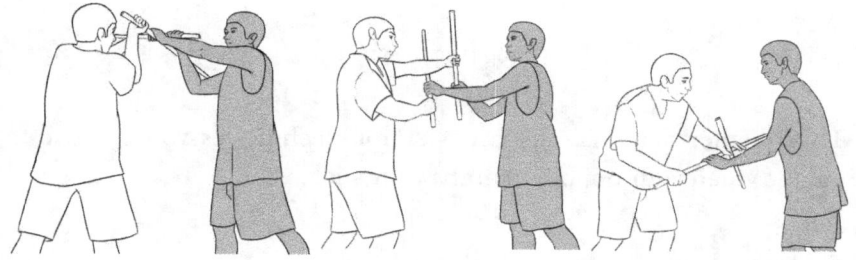

Related Chapters:

- Queen Strike
- Grab and Strike Drills
- The King of Strikes

BREAK-OUTS

This chapter demonstrates a few simple techniques you can use to escape when your opponent grabs your stick.

Butt-Thrust Breakout

This is a good option for when your stick is more horizontal than vertical. It makes use of butt strikes (strikes made with the bottom of your stick), which are extremely effective in close combat. Use your right hand to pull your opponent's wrist towards you as you thrust the butt of your stick into his torso.

You can also do this without the thrust to the torso. From this position, you can go into a simple arm-break and/or butt-strike combination.

For the arm-break, pull his wrist back toward you with your left hand as you apply forward pressure on his elbow with your right arm.

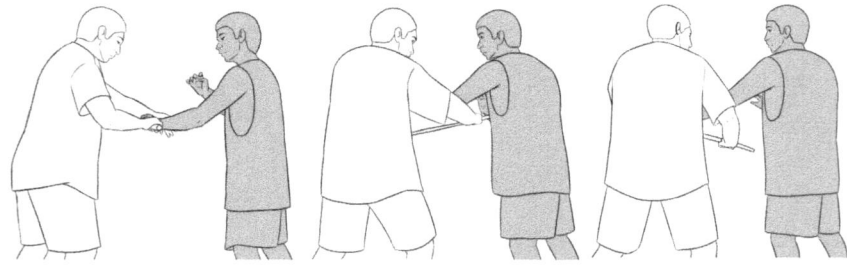

For the butt-strike combination, bring the bottom of your stick over your opponent's arm, hitting the side of his face with the bottom (the butt) of your stick. Slam your forearm down into the crook of his elbow to jerk him down, and then come back up into his jaw with the butt of your stick.

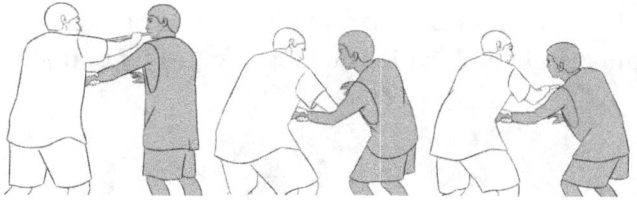

Elbow Breakout One

Use this technique when your stick is more vertical and your opponent has grabbed it, leaving little or no gap between his and your hands.

Bring the bottom of your stick up and in toward him, so your forearms are aligned and touching. Then slam the bottom of your stick/forearm down on his lower arm as you do queen strike to his head. This should be one smooth movement.

Move the bottom of your stick toward him in a vortex motion. By using a vortex, you move around his wrist, following the natural movement of his body. There is no need to fight him with force.

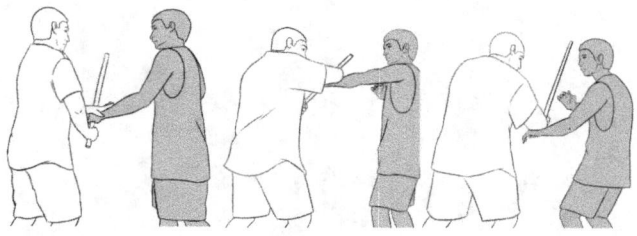

Elbow Breakout Two

A similar movement to Elbow Breakout One can be used no matter how big the gap between your and your opponent's hands is.

Grab onto either your stick or his wrist and then move the bottom of your stick over your opponent's arm in a vortex motion. Bring it down toward him and onto his arm. From here, you can do a queen strike or the butt-strikes combination, among many other options.

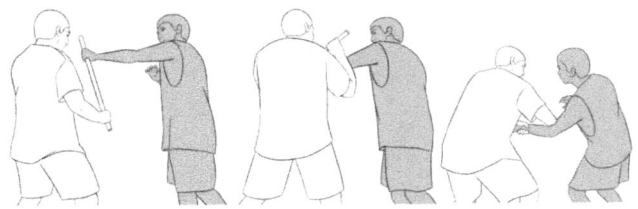

Related Chapters:

- Queen Strike

DOUBLE-GRAB SCENARIOS

When both you and your opponent grab each other's sticks, the person who knows what to do next and does it first will be the victorious one.

Gaining Advantage with Distance

When you're both at striking distance (or further), you're equal in terms of advantageous distance. When your opponent moves in and gets hold of your stick, it's bad for you.

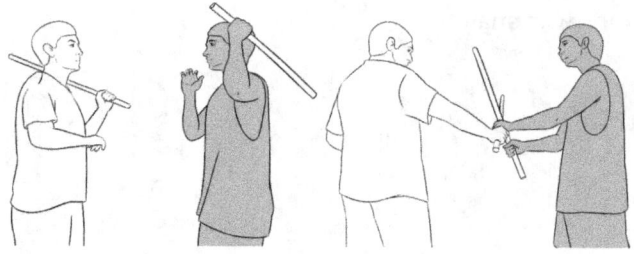

If you move in and grab his stick as well, then you'll be back to being equal.

The best position is to have your hand inside his guard. Amongst other things, it allows you to do the queen strike.

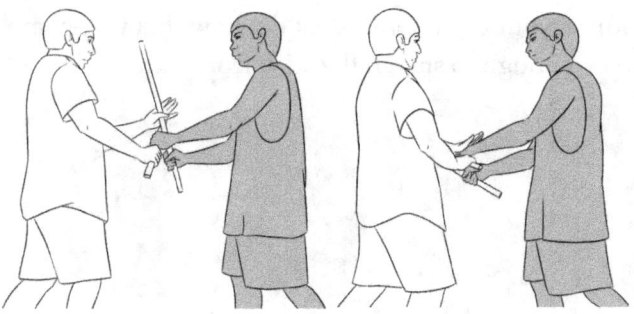

Double-Grab Adaptations

The same techniques that have been presented so far in this book can be adapted to double-grab situations. This chapter showcases a small number of these adaptations.

In these examples, you are the person on the left.

Hit-and-Twist Snatch

You both grab each other's' sticks in the high position.

Push towards your opponent with the intent of hitting him with the top of his stick. As you do this, change the grip of your left hand and do a hit-and-twist snatch.

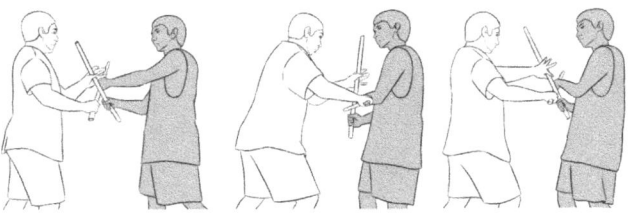

Twist-and-Hit Snatch

Your opponent grabs your stick high and you grab his low, with an underhand grip.

Pull the top of your opponent's stick down with a vortex motion. This will often be enough to snatch the stick from him.

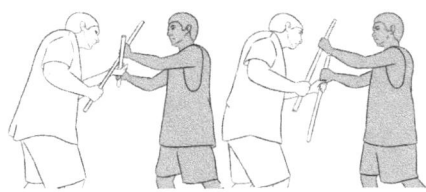

If not, smash the bottom of your stick down on his lower arm as you pull his stick up with your left hand.

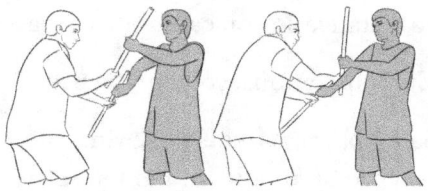

Fist Snatch

You grab your opponent's stick high and he grabs yours low.

Pull the top of his stick down and do a fist snatch.

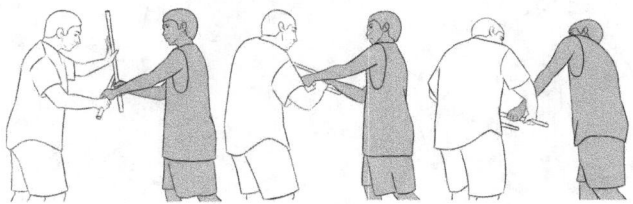

Elbow Breakout

You grab your opponent's stick high and he grabs yours low.

Bring your stick up and then slam your elbow down on his arm in a vortex motion.

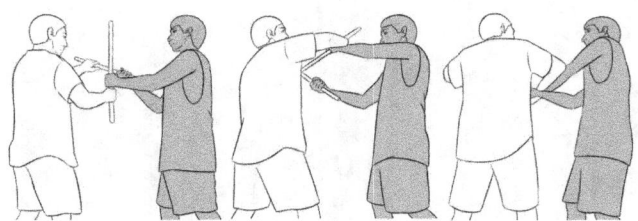

Returning to Seven

If you're the one in a disadvantageous position and get closed in on, you need to create distance so you can return to seven.

In the following demonstrations, you are the person on the right.

Step back to create space. As you do, bring the butt of your stick down. It is your arm that should straighten. Do not pull your stick back—you don't want to give up ground.

Once the butt of your stick is down, step forward again as you return to seven.

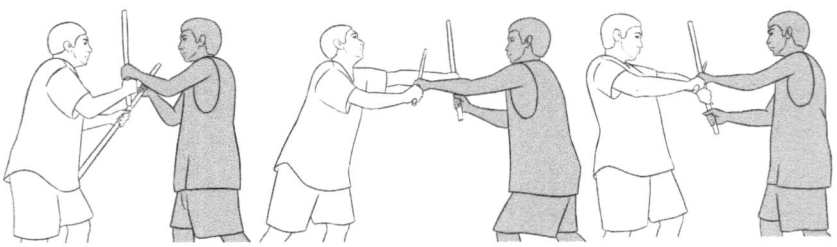

Double-Grab Countering Scenarios

The closing-in counter is a good move for when your opponent closes in on you.

As he does so, counter by putting your left elbow on his right fist and then twisting to your right.

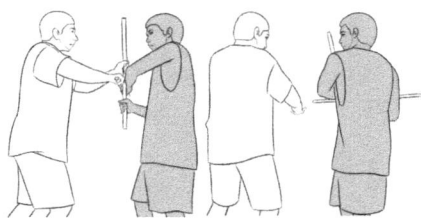

This demonstrates how you can counter the closing-in counter.

Hold each other's sticks in the high position. As you close in on your opponent, he does the elbow counter as previously described. Counter this by allowing the motion to happen and keeping hold of your stick, then pull up on your opponent's stick while smashing your stick into his hand.

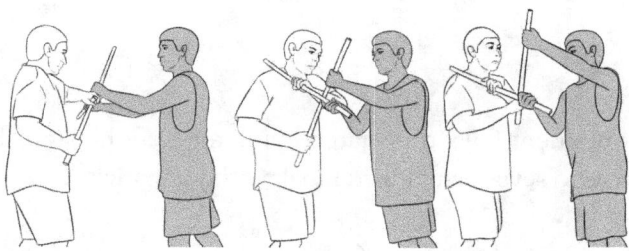

Push the top of your opponent's stick into his face so you can change grip and finish with a snatch.

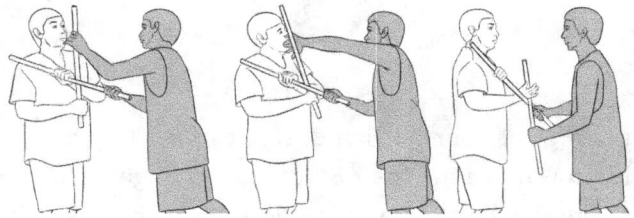

Double-Grab Drill

This drill is a good way to hone your reactions when you have hold of each other's sticks.

In this explanation, you are the person on the left.

Start with both of you holding each other's sticks and then begin to apply a fist-on-fist snatch to your opponent.

From the position shown in the first picture below, you need to push towards your opponent so you can change grip with your left hand

and then apply the snatch.

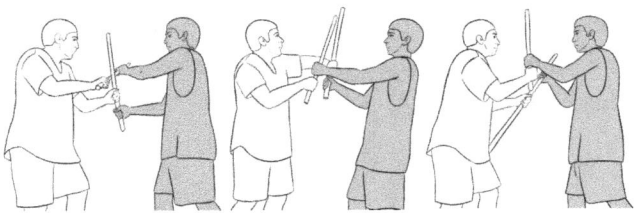

As your opponent feels the snatch being applied, he steps back and then returns to seven which you block with your stick.

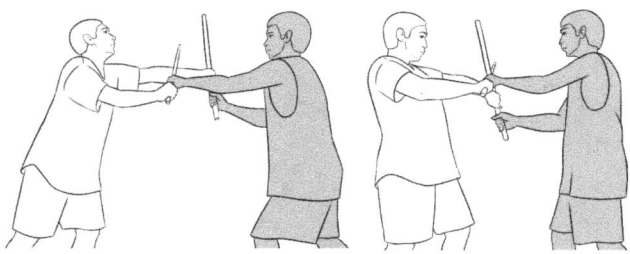

Change the grip of your left hand. Don't forget to push your opponent's stick towards him first. Since you changed your grip, your opponent senses what you want to do (that is, hit his arm with his own stick). To prevent this, he quickly moves his left hand to the outer side of your stick.

You change your grip again so you can apply a twist-and-hit snatch.

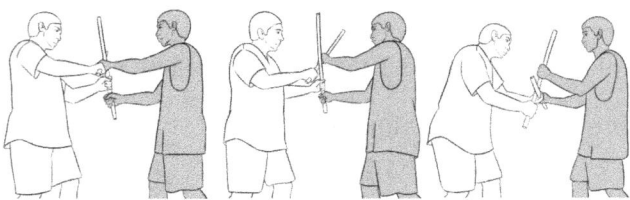

Your opponent feels it so he steps back and returns to seven, which you block again.

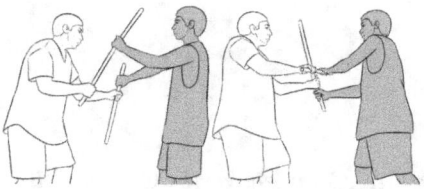

This puts your left hand in a bad position, so push towards your opponent and change your grip. Go to hit your opponent's left hand. To avoid getting hit, your opponent jumps to the other side of your stick.

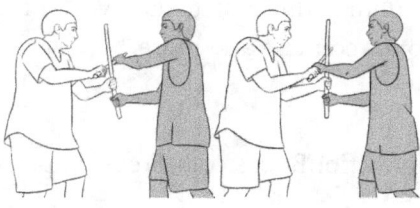

Change grip with your left hand and go for the fist-on-fist snatch to repeat the drill.

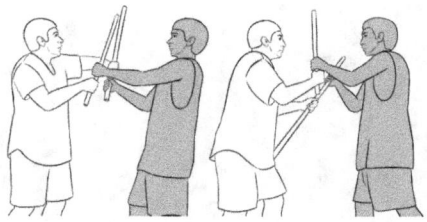

Once you and your opponent have gotten the hang of it, swap roles.

THANKS FOR READING

Dear reader,

Thank you for reading *Complete Vortex Control Self-Defense*.

If you enjoyed this book, please leave a review where you bought it. It helps more than most people think.

Don't forget your FREE book chapters!

You will also be among the first to know of FREE review copies, discount offers, bonus content, and more.

Go to:

https://offers.SFNonfictionBooks.com/Free-Chapters

Thanks again for your support.

REFERENCES

Abenir, F. (2014). *Eskrima Street Defense: Practical Techniques for Dangerous Situations*. Tambuli Media.

Anderson, D. (2013). *De-Fanging The Snake: A Guide To Modern Arnis Disarms*. CreateSpace Independent Publishing Platform.

Anderson, D. (2013). *Filipino Martial Arts - The Core Basics, Structure, & Essentials*. CreateSpace Independent Publishing Platform.

Anderson, D. (2014). *Trankada: The Joint Locking Techniques & Tapi-Tapi of Modern Arnis*. CreateSpace Independent Publishing Platform.

Buot, S. (2015). *Balintawak Eskrima*. Allegro Editions.

Cheung, W. (1852). *Dynamic Chi Sao by William Cheung*. Unique Publications.

DeMile, J. (1977). *Tao of Wing Chun Do, Vol. 2: Bruce Lee's Chi Sao*. Tao of Wing Chun Do.

Diega, A. Ricketts, C. (2002). *The Secrets of Kalis Ilustrisimo: The Filipino Fighting Art Explained*. Tuttle Publishing.

Godhania, K. (2012). *Eskrima: Filipino Martial Art*. Crowood.

Gould, D. (2016). *Lameco Eskrima: The Legacy of Edgar G. Sulite*. Tambuli Media.

Gutierrez, V. (2009). *WingTsun. Chi Sao II*. Sportimex.

Medina, D. (2014). *The Secret Art of Derobio Escrima: Martial Art of the Philippines*. Tambuli Media.

Paman, J. (2007). *Arnis Self-Defense: Stick, Blade, and Empty-Hand Combat Techniques of the Philippines*. Blue Snake Books.

Pentecost, D. (2016). *Put 'Em Down. Take 'Em Out!: Knife Fighting Techniques From Folsom Prison*. Allegro Editions.

Presas, R. (1983). *Modern Arnis: The Filipino Art of Stick Fighting*. Black Belt Communications.

Preto, L. (2016). *Multiple opponent combat: 10 lesson program with one handed weapons*. CreateSpace Independent Publishing Platform.

Wiley, M. (2011). *Secrets of Cabales Serrada Escrima*. Tuttle Publishing.

Wiley, M. (2015). *Mastering Eskrima Disarms*. Tambuli Media.

Yimm Lee, J. (1972). *Wing Chun Kung-Fu*. Ohara Publications.

AUTHOR RECOMMENDATIONS

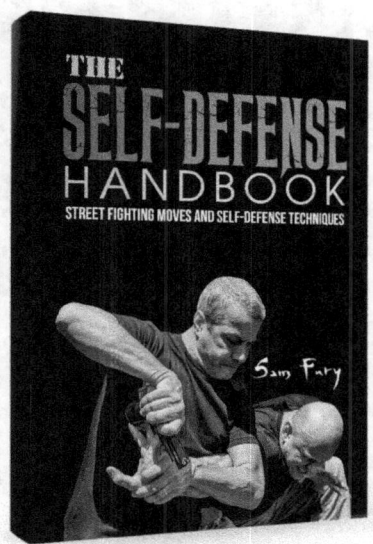

Discover all the Street Fighting Techniques You Need

Start learning what you need to win, because there ain't no rules on the streets.

Get it now.

www.SFNonfictionBooks.com/Self-Defense-Handbook

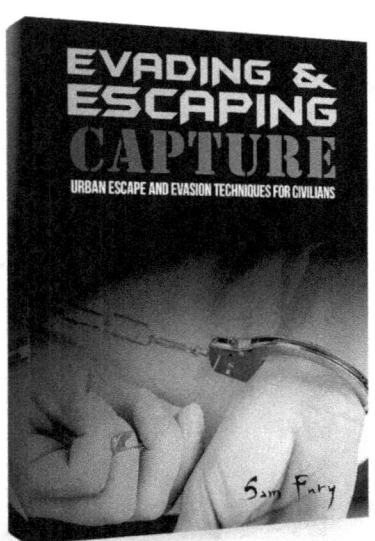

Teach Yourself Escape and Evasion Tactics

Discover the skills you need to evade and escape capture, because you never know when they will save your life.

Get it now.

www.SFNonfictionBooks.com/Evading-Escaping-Capture

ABOUT SAM FURY

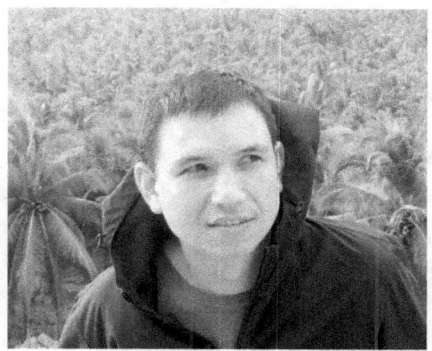

Sam Fury has had a passion for survival, evasion, resistance, and escape (SERE) training since he was a young boy growing up in Australia.

This led him to years of training and career experience in related subjects, including martial arts, military training, survival skills, outdoor sports, and sustainable living.

These days, Sam spends his time refining existing skills, gaining new skills, and sharing what he learns via the Survival Fitness Plan website.

www.SurvivalFitnessPlan.com

- amazon.com/author/samfury
- goodreads.com/SamFury
- facebook.com/AuthorSamFury
- instagram.com/AuthorSamFury
- youtube.com/SurvivalFitnessPlan

www.ingramcontent.com/pod-product-compliance
Lightning Source LLC
Chambersburg PA
CBHW071232080526
44587CB00013BA/1585